A Year of

(ME)

Mindful Eating to

Improve

Well Being

Printed in the United States of America

First Printing, 2017

ISBN 0-9994494-0-0

Royal Perceptions

RoyalPerceptions@gmail.com

www.RoyalPerceptions.wix.com

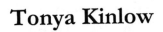

Tonya Kinlow

About the Author

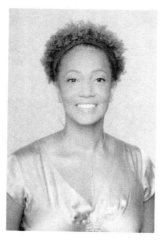

Tonya Kinlow is an excellent home cook who loves sharing creative, home-cooked meals with friends and family. In 2010, a major car accident involving her two children Evan and Taylor changed her life forever. As she contemplated life raising a child with a paralyzing disability, she shifted focus. Her focus shifted from fleeting materialistic goals, to how to follow a meaningful path, to health and wellbeing in the face of seemingly impossible barriers and daily hardships.

By 2014, Tonya married Chef Craig Stevens. It is safe to say that she has taken her passion for food and married it with her compassion for life. Self-described as "fairly healthy," Tonya has an active lifestyle, while not particularly athletic. She's a healthy eater, while not particularly small, and without subscribing to any single eating stereotype. Now with *A Year of ME*, Mindful Eating to Improve Well-Being, Tonya shares daily affirmations to bring awareness to living a well-rounded life. It is not a diet and it is certainly not just about food. It's about being mindful about how you approach life to reach your fullest sense of self. Since food is common to all of us, throughout every day of our lives, and for everyone we know, it is the most impactful place to make a change that benefits your entire life, in every aspect.

Tonya is not a doctor, nutritionist, or holistic leader. But just like you, she's been through some struggles and spent a lifetime focusing on weight and other self-attributes to complain about. In self-awareness, she understands that life's purpose is positive, not negative. She offers another way not just to survive, but to thrive one day at a time through mindful eating. Take precious time to focus on your strengths, not your weaknesses, and use your daily life experiences to lead you to overall wellness...mind *and* body.

Tonya is a food enthusiast and promotes compassion in sharing. She left her corporate career to start UGottaEat (UGE), an App Platform that gives unbounded access to *Homemade* and fresh-made foods which appeal specifically to your eating style...*On-Demand!*

UGE is dedicated to mindfully eating freshly made and homemade food for overall health, wellbeing, and happiness. Our social mission is to feed the world healthy foods while eliminating waste and food insecurity.

UGottaEat

Visit our Website at UGottaEat.com. Join our Blog to follow the mindful eating conversation, and Download the UGE APP to find homemade and fresh made food on-demand!

Follow Us & Join UGE at:

https://www.facebook.com/ugottaeatsomething/

https://www.instagram.com/u.gotta.eat/

https://www.twitter.com/ugottaeatsome

https://www.pinterest.com/ugottaeat

Dedication

To my love, Craig.

Acknowledgments

Thank you, Lord! Thank you, Universe! I am in a spirit of gratitude and giving the fullness of my thankfulness, to all that is. Nothing happens by chance, and so I thank everyone in my family and in my life. I understand that we are all connected. I understand that every encounter shapes me into who I am, and gives me the energy and direction for my next steps, to walk in my purpose.

This book was inspired on my way home after a Milestone Birthday trip with my best friends, who give me constant encouragement. Thank you, to Toi Jones and Marci Bennafield for providing inspiration and allowing me to inspire.

I could not have written this without the significant contributions and editing of Alexandria Cooper. She is a kindred spirit, super creative and full of light. Thank you, to Yehudhe Yehudah for editing and positive energy. A special acknowledgement to my daughter Taylor Campbell, for her encouragement, lending her face and energy to the UGottaEat brand as a beacon of light, her beauty, and exploration. Thank you to my son Evan Campbell, who inspires me every day and lets me know that we can create our own successes in spite of life's perceived roadblocks. I have the sincerest appreciation to Evan and his business partners Josh Schoeff and Ethan Hall for publishing A Year of ME.

Thank you to Caitlin Reynolds who helps UGottaEat in every way from events to the App as it grows and touches lives every day. Thank you to my parents for life, love and guidance. And finally, thank you to my husband Craig, who has given me the love, support, and freedom to follow my dreams, find my true purpose and pursue them.

Much, much love to all!

Table of Contents

Introduction

UGottaEat is dedicated to mindfully eating fresh made and homemade food for overall health, wellbeing, and happiness. This book is a compilation of daily affirmations devoted to improving your overall health by increasing your mindfulness through eating. Our social mission is to feed the world healthy foods, while eliminating waste and food insecurity.

You are what you eat. So, what are you today? Are you fried chicken and tempura vegetables? Maybe on your birthday, you're cake? However, on other days, are you the freshest food that God put on this earth for you? Be mindful!

A friend confided in me how she wasn't feeling well and said she hadn't eaten much. She had some cereal for breakfast and chicken liver for lunch. Where I saw an immediate correlation, she saw none. Organ meat has the sole purpose of filtering toxins of another animal. Processed cereals are full of chemicals, fats, and sugars that the body often resists, especially when topped off with dairy milk. The taste buds like it, so it can be a nostalgic treat from time to time, but its purpose does not imbue wellness.

When you don't feel well, assume it is for a reason. Something in your body is signaling a complication. Look at the clues and make a determination for things you can do to live healthily and not sickly. You don't need to be a doctor to do this. Awake your awareness. This book will encourage you to make informed choices to break out of low-energy ruts by eating well and ultimately, taking that new energy to make the best choices in all other areas of your life.

The choices are always yours and in front of you. There is no need for judgment. You are the master of your own fate. That is also the beauty of this book, enlightenment.

This book gives daily affirmations to lift you up in your journey to wellbeing. It gives practical reminders to pay precious attention to certain habits. It points out conditioning that we have experienced in our day to day lives that have inhibited our ability to live to our fullest. We begin to realize that we are making unconscious choices which leave us feeling down on ourselves. Then, we sabotage our own success. With *A Year of ME*, we turn this around on its head. We wake up to our greatest potential and our choices. We begin to make the choices that lead us to clarity, energy, and vitality. We begin to experience optimism and happiness. We do this one day at a time. We peel the onion back. We eat the elephant one bite at a time. (I do love a good cliché.) Patience. Patience. Patience.

I am patient. I am happy. I am whole. I am healthy. One day at a time. One meal at a time.

Think Differently—

This book will meet you wherever you are. It encourages you to think differently, find your uniqueness and celebrate it. It is okay to be a nonconformist in search of your purpose and to shed what burdens you. In keeping with this philosophy—

1) We share 366 days of affirmations to show a little respect for Leap Years! February 29th is also my birthday and extremely special to me. So, here's a quick fact that is learned in schools and then forgotten…

   It takes the Earth approximately 365 days and 6 hours to circle the sun. Our modern-day calendar has only 365 days in a year, so we add a leap day on February 29 nearly every four years to keep in alignment with the Earth's revolutions around the sun. Leap days keep us in alignment with the universe. It's a good sign.

2) This book is broken into seasons which don't necessarily follow the astrological dates. In this context, Spring is a season of renewal and awareness. Summer is a season of gratitude and activity. Fall is a season of intention and presence and Winter is a spiritual affirmation and purpose.

3) The first Daily Affirmation begins on March 1st which used to be the first day of the new year. Have you ever wondered why Sept means 7, but

September is the 9th month of the year? October through December following the same pattern.

When the calendar changed the new year by two months from March 1st to January 1st, the names of the months did not. We're going old school.

A Year of ME will shake up your thinking, allowing you to open your eyes to your infinite potential, which includes attaining happiness and wellbeing. For 366 days, I have carefully created inspirations to lead you towards the wellbeing of the body, mind, and soul. With these daily passages, you make an affirmation to yourself each day to better focus on your health – **physically** with what you eat and do, **mentally** with how you view yourself and others, and **spiritually** in how you fall into the flow of the universe.

Some days focus on diet specifics, while others allow you to let your imagination roam free. Some days might be difficult, while others could flow naturally. To venture out on a journey of wellbeing is no small feat. When you read these affirmations, you will be pushing forth through the darkness of doubt into the light of possibilities. Whether you read this book diligently each day of the year or freely flip through pages, allow these affirmations to act as the flashlight which illuminates your path. Each sentence read and each page turned, adds up to you actively cultivating a healthier being. And that dear friend, is an achievement to smile about.

How to read this book—

1. **Foundational:** Start on today's date and read one affirmation every day. Take time to think about the affirmation throughout the day. Read it more than once. Journal or talk to a friend about the affirmation to seal in the meaning and make it useful to you. Repeat it to yourself throughout the day. Allow it to marinate in your mind. Use it as a reference point for each thought and action.

2. **Accelerated Read:** Start on today's date and read 12 affirmations that correspond to today's date for each month of the year. This way you complete the book in 1 month. For example, if today is September 17th, read October 17th, November 17th, and the 17th of every month, thereafter. Acknowledge the similarities and differences of each affirmation.

3. **Topical:** There is an index in the back to cross-reference when you need specific encouragement on any given day. Need more awareness on eating? Could you use some encouragement? What about inspiration? Look in the index and find the topics. Then, read the affirmations specific to what you desire.

4. **Free-Spirited:** Read as many as you want, whenever you want, however often you want. Combine all the methods above and choose your own. Reinforcement and practice are key.

Your practice is awareness. Your practice is a path to happiness. Your path is unconventional. You by nature of your uniqueness are unconventional. Embrace that. It is a loving awareness that makes all other learning exciting. Keep a book at home and one at work or in your car. Use it whenever you need a little encouragement to feeling well. Get ready to wake up your thoughts and create a life of energetic wellbeing.

Spring.

March 1st

Today I expand my awareness.

It is inconceivable to know everything and all of the mysteries of the world. At the same time, it is wonderful to truly know this. To know, you cannot know everything. To know, the world gives us infinite opportunities to learn something new. To start again. To be fresh. You do this all, by expanding your awareness.

Pay precious attention to your surroundings. Take care of your wellbeing and increase your clarity. Learning and knowing more isn't exclusive to the resources of a library. Liberate yourself from that confining definition and you will open up to unlimited possibilities. You can know what it feels like to stand at the top of the Grand Canyon. You can know the freshness of a new day. You can know a storm. Each one is different. Each experience adds to your life when you take precious time to pay attention.

Today, expand your horizons. Expand your awareness.

March 2nd

I am eating purposefully.

I lose track of mindful eating at snack time. Not quite enough time has passed to eat, nor am I starving for a full meal. My grandmother called this desire to nibble or graze, being "peckish." This is where I typically fall victim to empty calories, where I fill my boredom with mindless chewing, tossing pretzels and cookies into my mouth without care.

The good news is I am eating purposefully now – and so are you. First, I recognize I *want* something. I truly don't have to have anything; but if I wait too long without making a decision or throwing something in my mouth, I might lose my resolve. My new detour for snack time is to make a smoothie for later and a cup of coffee for now. Throughout this expedition of mind, body, and spirit, I personally don't fancy regular coffee anymore. It's become a bit of a treat, my decaf cup topped with coconut cream (bonus points for no more caffeine addiction). Now I fill this want with the warm, comforting flavor of coffee. Small sips to remind me to take life slowly, appreciating the craft of the cup. I can now hold off until lunchtime to eat. I am eating and drinking purposefully, and damn, do I feel victorious!

March 3rd

I am renewed every day.

When we get bogged down in negative thoughts because of trying times and situations, we have to stop the spiral at some point and change the trajectory to take us to a positive place of victory. Claim a new vision each night before you go to sleep and reclaim it in the morning. Begin each day with a fresh Thank You, then set your intentions for the day.

Today will be better than yesterday. I will uncover the good in every situation and see what I want to see. I will forgive. I will be kind to myself. I will promote positive energy. I will have a superb day today, tomorrow, and the day after, with each morning a metamorphosis of change and renewal.

Simply, just breathe. Deeply. Once. Twice. Three times. Three times. I am renewed today.

"Do not conform to the pattern of this world, but be transformed by the renewing of your mind. Then you will be able to test and approve what God's will is – his good, pleasing & perfect will." -Romans 12:2

March 4th

I understand that my mind and body act as one.

When it comes to our weight, we steer the spotlight to our bodies – and that is where we miss the boat. Your weight starts in your mind and manifests itself in your body. Through this journey of achieving a healthy body, train your mind. Body and mind act as one, similarly to you and your significant other or any sports team. Individuals have different roles, but the team is one.

You are the one. Your mind is the quarterback or the center. Understanding this shifts your approach to wellness. The scale isn't really the barometer. Your mind's ability to focus on the positive, make healthy choices, and let go of thoughts that do not serve your awesomeness is the measurement.

Today, focus on your thoughts, not your weight.

"To keep the body in good health is a duty… otherwise we shall not be able to keep our mind strong and clear." – Buddha

March 5th

I make choices that improve my life one meal at a time.

We use food for comfort. We use food for entertainment. We use food as a respite from stress, anger, or sadness. We forget the purpose of food: to heal us and improve our life.

Control what you eat. Don't give your power to food. There is a popular saying, "don't bite off more than you can chew." Pushing each bite down and swallowing sweeter and fattier foods is an unhealthy route to feeling contentment or fulfillment. Most of the time we eat even when we have satisfied our hunger. Choose to eat mindfully.

By controlling your cravings and choosing smart meal alternatives, you'll unearth a newfound energy needed to make it through the day. It's awe-inspiring how many health benefits you receive from eating smart. You can run, jump, laugh, dance – whatever compels you to generate happiness. You can endlessly search for secrets to improve your life, but it all starts with the fuel we put into our bodies.

March 6th

I take responsibility for my life.

Everyone has those people in their lives that never take responsibility for their actions. When they're faced with an obstacle, it's the result of enemies or karma. Starting today, you are not one of those people. Think about times you blamed someone for your misery. Find your complicity in the situation and forgive them for your perceived injustice. Bring power and victory into your life through the force of forgiveness.

I knew someone who was unfaithful and blamed others for his divorce and misfortune. Because I believe in the Law of Attraction, there is a smidgeon of truth there. The larger truth is that he *was* unfaithful & dishonest – and that version of the Law of Attraction worked mightily in his life to his relationship's end. Remember: you own your decisions.

No one will fight your battles for you. When I have gone through difficult situations, I found that the answer was always within me. I took responsibility for my role in the dysfunction. Maybe not at the time, but I've matured. I've forgiven. Now I practice awareness for my choices and I take responsibility for me.

Live your life. Own it.

March 7th

Today I will choose the type of lifestyle I wish to live.

Back when I worked for corporate America, every project would take considerable effort to achieve the goal. Leadership encouraged taking control; "takes perseverance" they would command. With this motto ringing in my head, I would exert all my focus and energy on my workday. When I would finally arrive home, I felt spent. I left it all out on the field.

Give your energy to what makes you smile, what motivates you, or what brings you passion. When you have a goal to achieve, ask yourself, "what can I give to this project to make it a success?" What am I good at? What unique element of me can I breathe into this venture?

When you give freely, the best of yourself, the journey is easier and enjoyable. Give instead of taking. It blesses others and you. If that's not the type of job you have, find one. You'll be happier. You'll finally *enjoy* waking up for work in the morning. Find eating habits that give you energy the energy to follow your passions. Feed into meals that allow you to capitalize on this happiness. Perspective matters.

March 8th

I recognize that rest is an important part of vitality.

To sleep less than six hours is to deplete every possibility for success. Like water and clean food, it's essential to your wellbeing. Listen to your body. If you're tired, take a 20-minute nap. Anxiety, anger, & stress are directly related to lack of slumber.

More importantly, they affect more than just you. Quick tempers and impatience overwhelm your days and relationships suffer. The physical body needs rest. Think about your organs – brain, heart, kidneys – all require rest for better blood circulation to your extremities. It promotes thought and activity; without it we're delirious. Thought and activity are what lead to a character of wholesomeness. It's the well-rested person who extends kindness and compassion more readily.

Create a bed that welcomes you in each night, complete with the pillow of your choice and a blanket that reminds you you've reached home. Turn off the television, shut off your phone, and put away the electronics.

Nothing leads to increased vigor for tomorrow like a good sleep tonight; nothing is more fundamental than sleep.

March 9th

I am grateful.

Highlight this page. Hang it on your fridge. Frame it. Regardless of what you want to call forth in your life, gratitude is the miracle elixir that will make it appear.

A positive attitude produces positive results. When you are grateful, you cannot also be mad or negative. When you are grateful, you feel your body, your emotions, and you are present in the moment; it is your inner being opening up to receive goodness and grace, to receive light and love, to receive positivity.

Gratitude opens you up to receive whatever your heart desires. Do you want health and wellness? Peace? Happiness? Be grateful for what you have, as often as possible. Name things off one by one. Immediately upon listing your "thank-yous," you are met with the magic of hope; hope in the universe & hope in yourself. Whether you are thankful for something big, like the health of your family, or simply that the laundry is done when you come home from work, this gratitude keeps us constantly aware of our good fortune. And upon this awareness, we can fearlessly kick open that same door of opportunity. Be grateful.

March 10th

I am making a major change today to reflect my enthusiasm for higher wellbeing.

Do something wonderful today that illuminates to the world your courage to make the changes to live well. Try something new. Embrace the different.

Make an appointment for a new haircut. *Feng shui* the furniture around in your office or bedroom. Buy an outfit (or two) that expresses the style you want to have. Book a trip to that dream destination. Pick up that hobby you're dying to try. Book a spa day. Stroll around that art district you pass on your way to work. Sign up for a library card & check out a book. Call some old friends from back in the day and share some memories. Walk around the block. Clean out the garage. Go to the park and sit on a swing. Sign up for a 5K or half marathon.

Pick something. Anything. Something that resonates with you. Something that announces to the world it's a new day, and you're taking advantage of it. Break out into your greatness with a statement.

"The secret of change is to focus all of your energy, not on fighting the old, but on building the new." –

Socrates

March 11th

I am practicing patience because I know my dreams are manifesting as we speak.

I've stocked my fridge with vegetables, gave away processed foods, consumed a lake's worth of water, and squeezed more steps in - and still my clothes don't fit. But before I sulk in disappointment, I remind myself to be patient. Remembering it took time to take my body to where I am now, and it is going to take time to see positive results. When I stop my sorrows, and reflect on this journey, I will see my health is improving from each positive change I made.

Many people surrender when they don't immediately see results. It's the patient ones who succeed. Trust and know that when you practice healthy behaviors, you'll reap healthy results. It cannot *not* happen. Give the world, the universe, and the cells in your body time to move and rejuvenate to the awesome state that is building up energy, intensifying in fervor, ready to explode and present to you a magnificent body and spirit.

When it happens, it will be your patient perseverance that manifested your perfect health. The secret to success is patience. Today, I practice patience.

I am what I eat.

You are what you eat – you've heard this repeatedly throughout your life. From your mother who begs you to eat your broccoli, from the magazine articles you flip through, and even from your own internal monologue.

What you consume shows up on your waistline and on your skin. Your body is a window into your diet, reflecting each vitamin and mineral you absorb (or don't). Yet, it also appears in your attitude. If you eat poorly, you'll feel irritated and tired. But when you eat a balanced diet with a heavy focus on fruits and vegetables, your demeanor changes. You're genial, vivacious, and charismatic. If you are what you eat, then what do you want to gain from your food? What outcomes do you desire and who do you wish to be?

A clean diet means a clear mind. If you're looking for positivity, then eat well.

March 13th

I will satisfy my cravings with healthy choices.

Since cravings are essentially a cry for help, I will come to the rescue, cape flowing in the wind, spandex tights - the works. Here's my rescue plan:

First, I will think about why I am having this craving. Second, I will take long, deep belly breaths and close my eyes. Third, I will decide to either satisfy my craving or let it pass. Finally, if I decide to satisfy my craving, I will choose mindfully how I will do that.

If a craving is sweet, I can look to fruits and natural sweeteners instead of high-calorie choices. If a craving is for a crunchy food, I can bake vegetable chips, gnaw on celery, or slice an apple. If a craving is for fried food, I can find a baked alternative or choose pan-fried over deep-fried. If I want something creamy, I can have hummus or dip my spoon into yogurt. If a craving reminds me of someone, I will reminisce about the passing of time with an old friend.

You have an infinite amount of creativity and choices to confront before you choose to eat something that does not serve your wellbeing.

I am awake. I choose mindfully. I am my own hero.

March 14th

I plan what I will eat for the week.

You're less stressed when you have a plan. We set plans for travel, for our daily schedules, yet stop short of organizing our diets. Stop listening to people who complain of little time or hectic days. When you have a negative *outlook*, it is almost certain you will have a negative *outcome*. Simply decide. Painless. Practically effortless. It's easy to plan if you take the time to plan. You arrange many priorities without even thinking about it. Over time, healthy eating will be the same.

Do you plan to brush your teeth every day? Shower? Dress? Work? Of course, but it's become such a habit you don't think about it. When the toothpaste or toilet tissue is low, you plan to repurchase before you hit the cold cardboard roll. Do the same for what you will eat for the week. When you go shopping, start with at least three healthy green vegetables to have with dinners. Stock up enough for leftovers. Add three lean proteins. The rest is gravy. Plan the basics. The rest will follow.

March 15th

I bring loving attention to my heart today.

Thank your heart today. Otherwise known as the single most important organ in your body. No big deal, just some flesh keeping you *alive* and all.

How miraculous is the heart? This tissue that pumps every second of every day. It practically runs like a circuit board with electrical outlets, sending signals to your body to continue the flow of blood, contracting with each passing second. Each pump and squeeze control each process in your body. Most of us don't even think about our hearts until confronted with fundraisers for heart disease or if we see a heart-healthy icon on our groceries.

Place your hand on your chest and feel the drumming of each heartbeat. Lay your fingers on your neck and feel the blood rush through your arteries. This steady beat is the tempo of life. Love your heart today. It's employee of the year, with no days off. Ensure a strong, healthy heart by providing it with a clean diet and exercise. Celebrate your heart because it gives you life; that's no small feat.

March 16th

I practice mindful eating.

Mindful eating is dedicating time to pay attention and actively make choices. It is not a diet or restriction - it is liberating. You choose. You have the power over what you eat and therefore over your body and your health.

We've trained ourselves to eat like zombies. Have you ever mindlessly eaten potato chips? Then looked up, pulled your grease-coated fingers out of the bag, and said, "Dang, who ate all my chips?" This is a habit, and like all habits, it takes practice and dedication to break.

Start today and every day with a careful eye to break the bad habits that don't serve you. Start with the next meal you have, the next snack, or the next binge-watching marathon, and then practice. You think LeBron James rolls out of bed every morning and becomes "The King"? He wakes his skyscraper of a body up, heads down to the basketball court, and he *practices*.

Bless your food. Thank the cook. Smell the aromas coming towards you. Appreciate its nutritional benefit. See the spectrum colors. Determine what you will eat and eat mindfully. Repeat next meal for practice.

March 17th

I understand the path to success is paved with challenges.

Success is discovered through failure. This is a universal law, an expectation. From Albert Einstein to Bill Gates, people have paraphrased this rule over time, and you can determine the way to say it in the unique manner that resonates best with you. Maybe to you, it's known as impermanence, training, going through valleys to get to mountain tops, tearing muscles or breaking bones to come back stronger... whatever sticks in your mind best – just let it resonate.

Accept that life is not one straight rocket ship line to happiness wherein every single day you have exactly what you want. How boring would *that* life be? The adventure comes in the mistakes and the search for improvement. Understand that you obtain what you need, that the failures are simply the stops for gas along the cross-country route, so you can face these challenges with a "Bring it on!" attitude and a lightness that will propel you even further in your goals. Embrace the setbacks you meet as a necessary rhythm that's setting you up for your next success.

March 18th

I make decisions from positive emotions.

Positive outcomes are produced from positive thinking. It's that simple. Old advice like "don't go to bed angry" or "calm down before you go to bed" is widespread wisdom. The well-nourished and watered soil produces the best harvest and the most beautiful flowers.

When you make decisions out of resentment or from a bad attitude, you are not making the most positive decision. This decision does not come from your highest and best self - and it will not produce the highest and best outcome.

Your highest and best self, feel good. You smile when in this place or have happy butterflies and energy pulsing through you. Find this by closing your eyes, thinking about what fills you with pride. Linger. Notice your smile and emotion. Here is where you decide most assuredly. This decision, whatever it may be, will be the right one. Be well.

March 19th

I take three deep breaths when I feel upset and want a drink.

Every stressful moment, meeting, or long day leads me to say phrases along the lines of, "I wish I had a drink" or "I need a pint of cookie dough ice cream." Each spoonful of frozen yogurt and sip of red wine could act as barriers to avoid the problems at hand. When you fail to confront your honest feelings, and leave your emotions unchecked, you develop unhealthy habits.

Life will continually greet us with challenges. It is as natural as breathing. And it's okay. The world is not against you. On the contrary, the world is *for* you. Take a few deep breaths to remember this next time you're exhausted, overwhelmed, or distressed. You can make it through this on your own while building emotional strength. This strength brings you the power to take the good with the bad and the ups with the downs.

Take three breaths. Pour yourself an ice-cold glass of water or heat up a mug of tea. Stretch your limbs. Take a walk. Take back your health. Turn the down into an up.

March 20th

I humble myself.

When you hear someone telling you that they are humble, it's a warning sign. A humble person doesn't need to voice their humble nature, it is recognized through their actions and through their humility. The same is true for you.

Be yourself. Be honest and practice humility. The greatest acts of love and kindness are through service & compassion. It's tough to show compassion for others when you're too busy lifting yourself onto a pedestal. Find a way to look up at people in all conditions, not down.

Humble yourself.

"Humility is not thinking less of yourself, it is thinking of yourself less." – C.S. Lewis

March 21st

I am supported by others who enjoy a lifestyle of wellness.

Everyday, we have the opportunity to select good choices from bad. Sometimes without knowing, our friends can influence us during this selection process. We're familiar with the coworker who delightfully carries in the boxes of complimentary donuts each Friday. If you were approached with a dozen donuts, frosting glistening in the fluorescent office lights, would you grab one? Because they were right under your nose?

Sometimes, good people can occasionally act as poor influences. Take a step back from those who might seemingly look like good influences but might not be the best for your journey. There are positive influences around you who can lift you up and out of your donut daze. They will inspire you to try the veggie burger, to join them for a jog, and to live a healthier lifestyle a little every day

There is strength in numbers. Surround yourself with the positive energy you want to cultivate. The positivity of others will miraculously move its way over to you, and suddenly, you're not so worried about those donuts.

March 22nd

I will do something different today to shake things up and break my "habit" neuron pathways.

As humans, we fall into habits. You take the same roads to work, you eat the same quick meal for breakfast, and you sit in the same unassigned seat because that's become uniform to your routine. Our memory is wired to follow a distinct pattern.

A life of monotony is remarkably dull. Life is meant to be interesting. How incredible would it be to wake up each morning and have zero expectations for the day ahead? You could do anything you want – stroll around a museum for hours, try that new (slightly terrifying) exercise class, or attend a concert for a band you've never heard before.

Today, do something different. Quiet down the voice in your brain to turn up the voice in your soul. Break the routine. Walk the long way. Wear your most ostentatious outfit. Embrace the different and the strange, try something new. The further you venture into the unfamiliar, the more you explore what makes you unique and awesome. Break the habits today; if anything, it will at least be refreshing.

March 23rd

I take time to enjoy the color of the foods on my plate.

You eat with your eyes first. Generally, the more colorful your plate, the more nutrients you receive – and this excludes food dyes. There's nothing more boring or unappealing than a monotone plate.

Picture a plate with fresh country corn, bright orange carrots, and ruby red tomatoes decorating your entrée in the healthiest of ways. Notice how color affects you. The mood-altering properties of color can change your perspective from dim to hopeful. What's more enticing than a cherry tomato peeking out of the top of an emerald green salad?

Limit your distractions next time you sit down for a meal. Take the time to appreciate the bold colors of each ingredient. Acknowledge their power and their transformative characteristics. Smile because you're bettering yourself. Slower eating leads to better digestion, so take the time to take the time. Enjoy this bold plate; enjoy it with loved ones, co-workers, and yourself.

I love life.

This life is a gift, and what a wonderful gift we receive to walk upon an earth that gives us oxygen, the sun, and the rain. Each of us has parents, maybe a best friend or a pet that brings us comfort. Each of us has a place to call home. Each of us has the opportunity to better our lives.

Take precious time to today to love your life. Love isn't a textbook word with a definition you can easily look up. Nor is life. Love life. Those two words together create a massive existence. Then when you add "I," you have the most powerful sentence imaginable. Spend time with each word in that sentence. In its essence, loving life is a feeling, pumping with each heartbeat. This feeling draws upon an emotion that looks very much like gratitude.

While you reflect today on loving life, you are experiencing your best self. Spend time in a comforting environment that helps envelop a feeling of wellbeing. Eat well to nourish your body and spirit. Your life is a gift, and no, it's not sold at your nearest retailer. Don't re-gift it or try to exchange it for someone else's. Honor it. It is uniquely yours.

March 25th

My thoughts have the power to change lives.

We live on this earth together. With one another. We are an intricate, interwoven community and network of decisions & choices, consequences & reactions. Given this, your thoughts matter. You change lives. You can only be responsible ultimately for your own life, but you can and do impact others.

When someone confronts you with road rage or you enter the line of a cashier who clearly hates his or her job (or dealing with the public), you notice the energy. You feel the negativity. Luckily, the reverse is also true. When your thoughts are positive and you give someone a compliment or contribute to a good cause, it also is noticed.

This noticing is communication. You've been notified as surely as the pop-up notification on your phone or a message on your *UGottaEat* app - someone is reacting to your thoughts and choices. You are changing lives. Including your own.

March 26th

I will go to a fresh new market.

With chain grocery stores on every block, convenience has become paramount. A simple trip to the farmer's market on a slow Saturday yields a physical and a sensory experience. What better souvenir to take home from that food fair than fresh herbs and vegetables that are pesticide-free? Ones that still have dirt on their roots? The farm-to-table freshness makes every plate look appealing, bursting with color and flavor.

Preparing food in the kitchen without having to peel off a cellophane wrapper, toss out a plastic bag, or having to break out a brush to scrub off the preservatives is refreshing. There's something about connecting directly to the farm; there's a sense of community and reciprocity. It's an honest cycle, reflecting the circle of life.

"It's difficult to think anything but pleasant thoughts while eating a homegrown tomato." - Lewis Grizzard

March 27th

I recognize that the pain in my body is a call to action.

Pain is a siren cry from your body that something is wrong. That seems obvious when there is an open wound or blood, but we don't seem to think that way when you pull a muscle in your back or when you grapple with the constant cramping in your feet.

When you feel pain, notice it but don't dwell on it. Acknowledge that your health is misaligned. Then, self-medicate. Put yourself on a treatment plan, but not the one where you take a daily aspirin or old prescription medicine. Use food as medicine. It's the one thing that has a direct effect on your body that you take three times a day. An apple a day could keep the doctor away, but so could leafy greens and lean proteins.

Follow your doctor's orders, of course, and even your grandmother's home remedies, but incorporate what you now know to be true. Food is medicine, so tend to your pain wisely.

March 28th

Eating well + Awareness = Happiness.

A healthy body leads way to a healthy mind. A body that strengthens itself, defends itself, and loves itself is a gateway to an open-minded perspective. Good nutrition is the first link in the chain of wellness. When you eat better, you feel better. When you feel better, you function better – your body and your brain. High energy levels extend itself to preparedness and capability; a readiness to work, learn and experience.

Awareness is a tool for introspection, success, and peace of mind.

Eating Well + Awareness = Happiness. This simple equation is the only addition you need. Simplicity in general, whether it's on your plate or in your head, proffers clarity.

"My friend… care for your psyche… know thyself, for once we know ourselves, we may learn how to care for ourselves." – Socrates

March 29th

I wait 5 minutes and examine why I am having a craving and make a conscious decision.

It takes patience to practice mindful eating. Mindful eating isn't referred to as a spur of the moment decision. It's about pausing your initial instincts to create productive choices that will affect you positively.

Mindful eating involves a certain type of patience where you set aside a few minutes before each meal, snack, and craving to consider the food you're eating. You weigh its effect on your body & mind and how you can use that meal to improve your health.

Whenever you crave something, whether it's a slice of NY style pizza or a heaping pile of nachos, wait a solid five minutes before indulging. In that time, examine why you're having the craving and make a conscious decision. Improve your health one thought, one action, and one bite at a time.

I support local cooks and chefs who support my goal to eat well.

If you've ever worked in a restaurant, you've met your fair share of chefs. They might be strategically dropping curse words between each breath or they might be soft-spoken and gracious. Regardless, chefs bring a talent into this world not everyone holds.

The artistry of taste is one I admire. When I watch my husband cook, sifting flour or whisking egg whites, I am moved. As he cooks, eyes focused and wrists agile, he uses creativity to push me to eat better.

Support your local chefs who support your goal to eat clean, the ones who curated the special salmon salad and the ones who use few oils. By supporting these local cooks and chefs who are on a mission of wellness, you support your own mission of wellness.

A recipe for a healthy life: -1 cup of motivation

-3 tablespoons of creativity

-1/2 cup of willpower

-A dash of fitness and a sprinkle of support

Mix and bake until golden. Finish with the thick, sweet syrup of self-love.

March 31st

I choose abundance.

***

Your words and thoughts matter. They impact the outcome you are trying to achieve. The world would have you believe there are limited resources, that there can only be one winner, one President, or one Queen Bee. While it is true there may be only one titleholder, it does not mean that you will not hold those titles in the space that is meant for you. It does not mean you are not already perfect in who you are. Choose an abundant mindset. Create your reality. Lack begets lack and abundance begets abundance.

I have a friend who adopted a habit of running and (like me) runs at a slow pace and does more endurance races like half marathons. She collects medals not for running the fastest, but for finishing. She gains pride from these medals. Now, she's started her own trend, one that's evolved into a style: by entering single races, plotting a course, picking a date, and registering with an organization. You set that timer, shoot off the starter pistol, and – *voila* – she gets another medal. This friend of mine has an abundant mindset. Create your own success story. Invent a style that works for you. Make your own wins.

April 1ˢᵗ

I choose joy.

Sometimes it's hard to start up your day, isn't it? Like the Monday morning blues or the first day back to work after a vacation. Maybe it's the anniversary of the death of a loved one or a newly minted divorce. We all have these days.

When you feel overwhelmed from a day like this, take three long, deep breaths with your eyes closed and say today's affirmation, "I choose joy."

Follow this phrase with actions and gifts to honor you and this journey of wellbeing today. Today, treat yourself to a luxurious latte, start to plan a vacation, book a massage, steal a much-needed nap or fall asleep early. Choose things that give you something to look forward to – that give you hope. That will take the edge off the top.

Now to really get rid of the butterflies in the stomach and the tightness in the chest, delve deeper to your true self. There is deep abiding joy in all of us when we peel back the layers. Allow 15 minutes of quiet. Find your peace. Choose joy.

April 2nd

I make the conscious choice to drink alcohol only when I have pre-planned my eating choices.

Alcohol signals commemoration. Maybe it's for a life-altering event like a wedding or celebrating the end of a rough day. Whatever you're lauding with your glass of wine or craft beer, make the conscious choice to drink alcohol only when you have pre-planned your eating choices.

Oftentimes, we're greeted with a surprise night on the town, only to be led to a night spent in search of pizza. If you plan to drink alcohol at some point this week, set a condition of health. Maybe you only attend a party after you've eaten your allotment of vegetables for the day or hit up happy hour after you've reached 10,000 steps. Whatever it is, plan your healthy choices so you can consciously choose to drink alcohol. And always remember to stay hydrated. Supplement each drink with a tall glass of water and avoid that gnarly morning after migraine. Bonus points for jumpstarting your metabolism through the healing powers of hydration. Choose consciously. Drink thoughtfully. Eat mindfully.

April 3rd

I am visualizing my success.

With the ease of technology, we can guide ourselves towards our personal ideals of health. When you see someone who has the look you want, see it for yourself. Put your face on that body. Imagine a stronger, healthier version of you. Attach that ideal to your spirit. There's no need to hate someone else's positive attributes. Rather, allow them to positively influence you, learn from their challenges, and aim for an all-encompassing vision of health. Take a moment to adore them and send a quiet blessing.

This applies to the perfect job, the relationship you desire, and anything else you want for your happiness. Whether you see it in someone else or have an original thought, take time to imagine it's already yours. Daydream about it. Foresee a future you.

If you really want it, hold on to the thought. Ponder it every day, twice a day. Visualize it. Craft a vision board or put a daily reminder on your phone. You cannot achieve what you don't see. You can have what you put your heart and mind to. Visualize your success today, for tomorrow.

April 4th

I am aware that snacking after a meal is a habit I can break.

Many evenings, we finish a fantastic dinner and no sooner than we clear the table and dishes, do we start snacking. While you might opt for dessert, I opt for popcorn or nuts. There's something soothing about that hand to mouth oral fixation.

I am aware that this is a habit; and like any habit, it can be broken. I can retrain myself to adopt healthier habits, replace the bad with the good. And so can you. First, develop a recognition of your snacking habit. The next time you find yourself eating within an hour after dinner, remind yourself, "I am snacking out of habit." Choose healthier alternatives.

"We are what we repeatedly do. Excellence then, is not an act, but a habit." – Aristotle

April 5th

I focus on my food while I am eating.

Focus on eating while you're eating. Keep the distractions at bay. When you drive, just drive. When you study, just study. When you're doing emails, just do emails. Anything you do with your full attention, you'll do it better.

Multitasking is a strategy of quantity over quality. Choose to make quality decisions in your eating to focus on your outstanding results of those quality decisions. Your food will taste better and be much more appreciated. You can close your eyes after you've taken a bite to really mingle with those flavors in your mouth. Feel crunch and the smooth; taste the sweet with the savory.

Focus on your food. When you eat, eat.

April 6th

It is my intention to be healthy.

What does health look like to you? Are you fit and toned? Do your clothes fit loosely? Is your posture taller? Are you able to walk a little further? Whatever it looks like for you, see it. See it in your mind's eye and know you will achieve that state.

While strolling down the street, I bumped into an old friend whose appearance left me speechless – her overall presence amazed me. As we were chatting, I scanned her face, attempting to pinpoint what changed. She glowed, smiled wide, and eyes brightened with enthusiasm as she spoke. I asked if she had lost weight and she replied with a passionate yes. She admitted her doctor revealed she neared a pre-diabetic state; clearly, she heard the warning shot. She altered her diet and started exercising – a simple recipe for a profound feeling.

When I look in the mirror now, I remember how lively I felt her energy and spirit. I remind myself, I'll soon be like her. It is my intention to be healthy. I intend to journey down this path of wellness to gain the energy of pure sunshine and the spirit of my youth (the compliments I'll take, too).

April 7th

Today I focus on foods that make my body feel good.

Today's technological age steadily saturates us with news, updates, and social media. It transcends from our smartphones to our daily diets, where we have information overload on what is the right way to eat. Spend time thinking about what works for you. No one knows your body like you do.

What makes you feel bloated or itchy or breaks your skin out? Avoid that. What foods influence you to want to take a mid-day nap? Take a pass on that. Pay attention. Experiment. Do your own research based on your body type. You can read articles galore on what's beneficial for your health or age group, but only you will know what empowers you (or what puts you to sleep).

We believe certain conditions are hereditary. If our parents or grandparents had this and that, then we will too. Only a small percentage of heredity is passed through your genes; the rest is a personal experience. You can change what your parents, grandparents, and great-grandparents did – you can change by choice. Focus on foods that give you energy. Break free from your hereditary confinements. Your wellbeing is worth it.

April 8th

I wait 5 minutes before I satisfy a sweet and salty craving.

Salt-based and sweet tooth cravings are mostly based off of habit. The habit of indulgence and regularity in your diet – like clockwork after your carb-filled feast or that nightly cookie. Both salty and sweet cravings link directly to the neurons in your brain by releasing serotonin, similarly to the effects of drugs and alcohol.

My method of avoiding hankerings, in general is not to skip meals. I notice when I forget my morning yogurt, I compromise with myself to splurge. Skipping breakfast could lead you to overcompensate later in the day to the point where you'll eat anything simply to feed yourself. And that's where those dreaded salt-or-sweet cravings arise; you grab the candy bar at the checkout because the salad bar is on the other side of the store.

However, if you accidentally skipped a meal or truly need to fulfill that craving, opt for healthier choices. If you want toast, switch it over to a quinoa salad. Donut? Try a smoothie. Burger? How about a salmon patty? No matter what your craving is, there is always a healthy option that will suffice it while being guilt-free.

April 9th

I thank my body for carrying my mind through the day.

Our beliefs create our thoughts. Our thoughts create our actions. Our actions create our reality. Our mind is at the center of creation. Too often do we find a way to negatively view the world, our own body, or others – and we see the result through tragedy-stricken news channels or celebrities teaming with surgeons to design the ideal body image.

Change your thinking. They are *your* thoughts. You actively control them with patience and practice. When your mind says you feel lousy, take time to examine why you think that. Look beyond the surface of "my belly is hanging out" or "this is not what models look like on magazine covers." When you start to look for the good in situations, in people, and in life, you will find it.

Reclaim your own beauty. Inner *and* outer. Your belly does a great job, and so does the rest of you: at holding that mind in your head, at fueling your workday, at allowing you the energy to wake up with the rising sun, at giving you the opportunity to feel the wind on your face. Thank God and thank the universe for your functioning, beautiful body.

April 10th

I understand that others' opinions are a reflection of them and not me.

Judgment is based on self-perception. When people see their perceived flaws as perfections onto someone else, there's this heightened need to analyze these flaws. For instance, toned muscles, bright smile, or sharp wit is nice. But fixating and comparing these characteristics and tearing others down to make yourself feel better is unhealthy.

The opinion of others directly reflects their insecurities. People manifest their personal insecurities onto others in order to feel better about their flaws. If someone calls you stupid, it's because they themselves are insecure about their intelligence, and they want to make themselves feel smart. Know that opinions have nothing to do with you, but everything to do with who states that opinion.

If you face a bully or hear someone talk poorly behind your back, know that this is a sign of their character. Tune out the negativity from others to turn up the positivity in yourself. Love yourself; it'll drive them crazy.

April 11th

When I let go, I gain everything.

We change every day. Each time we open our eyes, we establish new ideas and shift our perception. Yet, we hold on to old thoughts about ourselves and other people. Have you ever experienced the power that stems from forgiving others? Forgiveness is the best kind of selfishness. It is self-indulging because it makes your life boundlessly better. Every enemy we forgive; every forward step we take or every bite we chew – all shape our future in the next moment.

Think about how different you were 10 years ago. Now consider how different you were five years ago. What has changed in the past year of your life? Six months ago? Last week. The last 20 minutes. When you know that life is constantly changing, you release past hurts, negative impressions, or body image barriers. You gain opportunity, more love, and more acceptance; you gain the things you want when you let go.

What will you do today to let go? Will you abandon comparison once and for all? Will you finally beat up the bully in your life? Will you forgive? You choose everything in your life. Choose tranquility, health, and happiness.

April 12th

Today I bless my waistline and give thanks for the early warning signs it provides me.

Waistlines are the butt of many complaints. Poor waists are stuck with a poor reputation. For centuries, they were squeezed into corsets. In the last decade, they've been altered by plastic surgery with the commonality of free toothbrushes at the dentist. When we lose weight, we focus on our abs, hoping it'll whittle our waist.

Lay off the waistline today. Quit it with the complaints. Your waistline is a blessing. Give thanks for all it does for you. Your mighty waistline reveals your lifestyle; it quietly informs you of your progress on this wellness journey. An inch gained could mean you need to tighten your focus, while an inch lost means you're on a victorious path. Show some love to your unfairly criticized waistline today. It balances you in more ways than you think.

April 13th

I have a positive relationship with food.

Food is critical to life. It is the basic building block. No one can survive without food. It is the most important relationship in your life. If you are fortunate to eat three or six times a day, you already make up a small percentage of the world that can eat without worry or without fear of tomorrow. While you enjoy your fresh produce and clean water, there are those who go hungry, who are food insecure, who don't know where their next meal will come from.

Take time to think about how food sustains you. Give thanks. List three things about food that you are thankful for. What makes you happy about food? Abandon those negative food choices that bloat you and inflame your body with artificial products and trans fats. Trade them in for the snacks that soothe your stomach and entrees that energize. Nurture a relationship with food that sustains you. Eat leafy greens every day, drink two liters of water, and discover your sugar cravings in the freshness of fruits.

Food gives you life. Good food gives you a good life. It's an important relationship. Pay attention and honor the intimacy.

April 14th

I choose portion sizes that align with the level of health and wellness I desire.

Pick portion sizes that will reflect your wellbeing. Our eyes are often bigger than our stomachs and size can be deceiving. You load up a hefty plate, but you realize halfway through you're full. Most of us take it as a challenge and eat not because we're hungry but because it's in front of us, beckoning our attention through color, smell, and taste.

Portion sizes help you to find clarity in your diet. Cutting back on your heaping plate can fulfill your taste buds without overfilling your stomach. Having a little bit of everything isn't nearly as bad as having a lot of everything. If you're out to dinner or at a friend's dinner party, scoop up some of those buttery mashed potatoes, simply don't allow it the authority to take up the whole plate.

Life is meant to be enjoyed, so try what you can - just in small portions. With small portions, you're in control. Take back your diet, one scoop at a time.

April 15th

I recognize that anything worth having is worth waiting for.

Anticipation can be so much fun if you let it. Remember looking forward to holidays, birthdays, and the last day of school? If these things happened every day, they wouldn't be so special.

Recognize the things that have taken precious time to manifest or reveal themselves. Aren't those the most rewarding? It takes experiences more than time. Time is a measurement on a clock or a calendar. What really makes up life, are your experiences.

Pay attention to life and slow down. Stop with the fast food and experience the slowing of time while cooking with family. Eat a meal at the table with actual plates. Skip the drive-up ATM at the bank; park the car and walk in to interact with others. These seem simple. Life becomes much richer when you experience it. Don't let it pass you by.

April 16th

Homemade = Happiness

___

There's an indescribable ingredient in homemade food that's not found in your average restaurant. It's the moments spent with family, rolling out dough to make scratch made pasta. It's those glorious mornings spent alone as you softly crack eggs and slowly slice vegetables for an omelet. It's the dinners spent with your significant other as one of you work on the entrée while the other works on the appetizer. It's love, and you don't find love at every drive-thru window.

It's the time you spend with the food that matters most. Those minutes or hours, even days, where you mull over ingredients to create a meal birth a satisfaction from your dedication. You create a relationship with your food as you slice and dice, sauté and bake. In that relationship, you discover peace and happiness. And when it's spent with family and friends, those feelings only multiply. It's love.

April 17th

I adopt the habits of people that surround me.

We are influenced by our surroundings. Our actions are often a reaction to something else, whether it is a force of nature or the peer pressures of friends. No matter how strong or independent we fashion ourselves, at our core we are simply energy. Like a magnet, we attract and repel. Today, administer special attention to who exist in your daily interactions and note the habits that they hold.

Awareness of what encircles you will allow you to see yourself more clearly. We all are connected; some scholars theorize we are all the same. You do not live in a vacuum. You influence others just as they influence you, often unknowingly. Your thoughts, opinions, and habits are influenced by who's in your circle – so pick a team of all-stars.

Do they lead active lives? Eat healthful foods? Or do they brag about their couch potato afternoons or frequent nearby bars and fast food restaurants for most of their dining experience? Consider how the habits of others affect yours. Increase your awareness so you may shape your own experiences and create your own way of life. Surround yourself purposefully.

April 18th

I am aware that my thoughts control my emotions.

Start noticing your actions in the present moment. When you mindlessly eat a bag of potato chips, what were you thinking about? Probably not the chips. Were you watching a movie, reading, or even driving?

Your thoughts guide your choices. Your choices guide your thoughts. It becomes a happy dance, but it has to start with the first step and attunement to the melody. Be aware of your thoughts. You actively select your thoughts just like you choose which route to take to work or what to wear. Choose positive thoughts. Then, choose the right action to achieve your best health.

Think healthfully. Choose healthfully. That's when you will be healthy.

"In the mind is everything. What you think you become." – Buddha

April 19th

I am making at least one conscious choice to avoid processed food today.

Healthy people have to be label readers. Processed food comes in many disguises. Until you read the nutrition facts on the side of the product, you can easily be fooled. Dangerous nitrates, sulfates, and chemicals I don't dare pronounce are often part of the small print packaging - if you can't pronounce it, don't eat it.

It's no longer simply food dyes and pesticides; it's scientists breeding genetics to modify your food for eye appeal and taste. Giant letters on the packaging, which scream "Non-GMO" or "gluten-free," can be defeated by these chemical infusions that put taste ahead of health.

Explore beyond boxed and packaged foods. Stop by your local farmer's market. When foods don't have a label of nutrition, simply ask the grocer. Be your own health detective.

April 20th

I am balanced.

Awareness is key. Everyone hears tips and tricks, adding to their self-perceived credibility on how to be healthy. Yet, they do not do what needs to be done to have a life full of wellness.

Become aware of balance. Balance in all areas of your life comes from becoming aware of your confidence and sense of self. We lose doubt to discover wholeness.

One key area of awareness is in your health. Eating processed and fattening foods consistently result in sickness, sometimes even irreversible disease. Everyone knows this. There is no magic pill to aging, weight loss, or good health. The solution is balance. Focus on caring for yourself. Attract abundance and do not focus on lack. Nurture your personal growth and achieve balance.

"In order to carry a positive action, we must develop here a positive vision." - Dalai Lama

April 21st

I am aware that sugar is addictive.

Sugar chemically produces endorphins. In that sense, it's like a drug; it produces endorphins in the brain that give you a feeling of satisfaction and a need for more. The candy bars and chocolate drops are visually appealing. But sugar shows up cleverly disguised as orange juice, flavored waters, dairy products, cereal, and even lip balms. And this only increases our desire for more. Like anything addictive, sugar is a craving.

Have you ever eaten one piece of chocolate? Or chewed one gummy worm? Like a drug, there's a ritual around sugar. We resort to sugar after rough days to console us, after dinner to complete our meals, and in the middle of the afternoon for a quick sugar high.

Do your homework. Find out where sugar hides. It goes by many names: dextrose, corn syrup, fructose, and xylitol. Know what you're putting in your body and how your body reacts to it. Know when to say no.

April 22nd

I feel good that eating well enlivens me and helps the environment.

Today, realize how your healthy eating means a healthier planet.

Eat local so you can cut back on gas emissions from food that travels hundreds of miles, leaving pollution in its path. This means grown and produced locally. If you have the option to pick out local produce, take advantage of that opportunity. You grow healthier while allowing the planet to grow healthier in return.

Eating well for you and the environment also means cutting back on red meat. For example, cows release methane gas, similar to the emissions from large trucks or cars. Cutting back on red meat means cutting back on the demand for red meat, and essentially cutting back on harmful pollution. Choose lean, local proteins instead like chicken, pork, or lamb. If you can, try out vegetarianism for a week.

Like a chain reaction, when you choose the locally sourced salad over the fast food burger, you create a wave of influence that saves the planet one leafy green at a time. Know your worth - individually, locally, and globally. You impact much more than the numbers on a scale.

I acknowledge that uncertainty is the natural state of life.

Life is unpredictable. You can never anticipate fate. There are expectations, of course, but the future is a mystery.

You will never foresee the future and you'll never truly be prepared for any issue. But, isn't that kind of amazing? That every single person in this world genuinely doesn't know what will happen tomorrow? A life where you planned out each second of the day is uneventful. If you did have the cliché crystal ball of the future, your life would lose that precious element of surprise.

Today, acknowledge that uncertainty is the natural state of life. Roll your shoulders back, lift your head up high, and put on a brave face as you conquer the uncertainty that is life. Life won't always proceed as imagined, but it's those unexpected moments that bring lifelong memories. Learn from them and grow.

April 24th

I am aware that excessive body weight can lead to chronic diseases.

We have been made aware of many of the chronic diseases that have exploded in our society. From diabetes to heart disease, to cancer. We hear about them, watch our family members struggle, and we often fear our own diagnoses.

Now we need to increase our awareness to the *causes* of these diseases. Turn your attention to preventing and reversing these diseases. Start today by eating a whole food diet for improved wellness. Excessive body weight is the result of eating foods high in toxins and ingredients that your body doesn't process well. Your body becomes clogged up and stores toxins instead of releasing.

Be aware. Eat good foods. Make chronic diseases obsolete. Prevention is key.

April 25th

I am visioning my life as I want it to be.

Think back to your teenage self. You might have been slightly awkward or constantly fussing with your braces. Remember your room? You probably tore out pages of magazines and plastered inspirational quotes, athletes you admired, or out-of-reach celebrity crushes to your walls. What was once your mother's favorite wallpaper transformed itself into a mood board of your hopes and dreams.

Visioning these idols and adhering inspirational phrases to the walls shaped your values. You would envision the person you wanted to be. Our walls were our vision boards. They gave us our daily dose of creativity. They inspired us.

Right now, vision what you want for your life, for your mind, and for your body. Write down the motivational quotes. Work a little bit every day to illustrate your life with positivity. Think of the universe as your bedroom – tear out the magazines, slap the stickers on your walls, and send out messages to the world around you that your life is positive. Extend your hopes and dreams past your bedroom walls. Extend them into the universe.

April 26th

Today I focus on fiber.

Fiber is usually linked to the toilet so it gets a pretty crappy reputation (c'mon, that was funny). Fiber keeps your digestive system moving by efficiently removing the waste from your body. But there are different categories of fiber: soluble, which lowers cholesterol, and insoluble, which keeps that digestive train on its tracks. By balancing these two types, your body normalizes your bathroom breaks and aids in weight loss.

High fiber foods fill you up and leave you satisfied longer, so you aren't running to the freezer post-dinner for ice cream. With a full stomach, you avoid the temptation to mindlessly snack because you already feel full. Some fibrous options can even lower your cholesterol through the absorption of cholesterol from your diet.

Today, focus on fiber. Acknowledge the effect fiber has on your dietary habits. Honor the role fiber holds in your body. Invite fiber on your journey towards health; it can keep you moving in the right direction.

April 27th

My motives for eating well align with my highest and best values.

We tend to focus on eating well as a way to lose weight. Whether it's for vanity's sake or under doctor's orders, it can take on the persona of a forced decision. Forced decisions do not provide lasting results. When you function under stress or against your will, you cultivate a negative energy and your effort will be hard, difficult, and laborious. That's why you quit so often and run for the supersized combo meal. Direct your attention to the value you desire and the right motivation will propel you to success effortlessly.

You desire energy, health, vitality, love, and happiness. With an active lifestyle and fresh take on food, you can have the energy to participate in the community or the clarity of mind to remember your Stepsibling's birthday. It all starts by making the best decisions for yourself and your life. Eating well will allow you to achieve that. One bite, one meal, one day at a time.

Before you know it, your clothes will fit how you want them to and your doctor will be happy to only see you once a year for the annual checkup. Elevate your motives and success follows faithfully behind.

April 28th

Gratitude allows me to have compassion for others.

Times have occurred in my life where I was unusually caught up in my own problems, I could not give any compassion to others. (Misery really does love company - it's true!)

Compassion brings sunshine into lives of darkness. It quietly whispers love into empty hearts. When you notice a negative person, offer encouragement and compassion. These people need compassion the most; have they lost their sense of direction, their motivation, or their happiness?

Stay alert to avoid the contagion of a negative spirit or personality. Your emotions come from within *you*. No one controls your emotions but you. Don't be influenced by the negativity of your peers, but be influenced by the positivity of your leaders.

When you include compassion in your mindset and see clearly what others endure, gratitude follows closely behind. And it's a cycle. My son is in a wheelchair. I can't tell you how many people have been inspired by their compassion for him and thankful for their own capabilities. Choose the positive cycle. Compassion... rolls off the tongue, doesn't it?

I eat well to have energy for my friends.

There are days where I look forward to nights spent relaxing on the couch. You grab your favorite magazine or book and your coziest sweatpants for a night in with yourself. But is there anything more conflicting than when a friend calls you up for an impromptu adventure when you've already sunken into a couch cushion?

I find I crave these lazy days when I eat unhealthily. After consuming whatever junk food, I chose, I beeline to the living room. When I eat well, however, I have energy for my friends. I desire to paint the town red. I have a vigor for life that provides me with the endurance to chat ears off and dance the night away.

If you don't have the energy for your friendships, you miss out on the relationships that give you happiness, laughter, and support. Seize the day and call up some friends. Slip in a salad beforehand to give you a clean energy. If you want to maintain your relationships, you need the energy to do so.

Eating well isn't only for you - it's for others, too.

April 30th

I practice non-resistance.

There are things that happen in our lives that we just don't accept as real or true. Denial can be destructive and cause us to do and show destructive behaviors. Practice seeing a situation for what it is and not resisting it. No need to push against a brick wall. Acknowledge the wall that exists in front of you and plan accordingly. Walk around it if you must. Climb over it if you can.

Accepting things as they are, does not mean you approve of them. It does, however, allow you the clarity to take the best and highest action appropriate for your wellbeing. Don't resist your boss, spouse, or the current state of affairs. See things as they are. Don't resist the truth staring you in the face. Accept it and then you will be free to choose the best course action.

Find your freedom. Practice non-resistance.

May 1st

Now is my time.

The past has passed and the future is far: be present. Stay in the moment when you grow bitter about a past hurt or anxiously wait for the future. All we have is now and in this moment, there is no issue. In this moment, you are reading this affirmation, you are turning the pages - you are alive.

The author Eckhart Tolle, in his novel, "The Power of Now," inspired me to stay in the present to move past a difficult period in my corporate career. I disagreed with my boss's ethics. While the threat of losing my job was real and my fear profound, my extreme reactions to stress and headaches added no benefit to my life. I only found peace by practicing presence, living in each moment and taking the steps, I needed to quit. I worked my butt off, interviewed with other companies, and made my way out of the darkness with my head held high.

Everything passes; life goes on.

Pay attention to now. Be present. Don't wait until tomorrow to eat healthily or join a gym. Don't wait until you get to a certain weight to start dating or get married. Or to book your dream vacation to that sublime island. You are you right now. Live. *Now* is your time.

May 2nd

I keep healthy food choices handy.

What's in your refrigerator, pantry, car, and purse? Do you have candies, cookies, and chips equipped for cravings? Replace those processed items with natural or organic snacks that will revive your health and wellbeing.

Examine those moments in your daily routine where you fall short of your snacking potential. Is it after your morning cup-of-Joe? Is it before you head home? Is it right around the time you ready for bed? Stockpile on choices that will enable you to reach your goals, and set them up for the future to ensure a path of positivity.

Stash a bag of heart-healthy walnuts in your car for those rush-hour drives. Have some kale, apple, or banana chips for when you crave a snack with some crunch. Keep a fruit bowl on your desk at work for your late afternoon sugar fix. Share with your colleagues and invent a new work ritual. Share with your friends. Share with anyone who could use a nutritious boost.

The quality of the foods you keep around you is directly correlated to the quality of your health. It's time to re-think and re-stock. What's in your kitchen?

May 3rd

I am consistent.

Start your days by asking yourself the question, "Who am I?" Sit with the question. Dissect your answer. Over time, you will initiate this conversation more willingly as you begin to know yourself so you can *be* your best self. There's consistency in who you are. Pull it out of your inner knowing.

Your wellbeing is nurtured with one good choice after another. Aim for consistency. When you stumble, promise to continue on your course. Self-correct. Soon your good choices outweigh the unhealthy choices. You will become happier and happier with your results day after day.

Who are you? In this moment? Who were you yesterday? Who will you be tomorrow? Who are you? Are you friendly? Then be kind to yourself. Are you striving to be healthy? Then grow into that person through your choices. Consistently.

Who are you... consistently?

May 4th

I recognize that the culture of eating out promotes large servings.

Pay attention to the serving sizes at restaurants. What is labeled a meal for one could easily satisfy two people. If you head down to that family-owned restaurant, you'll encounter family-style plates, a serving platter intended for a family of five. As picky eaters during our transformative years, we were taught to clear our plate and not waste food. So, when we go out, we eat way too much; with our parents' voices ringing in the back of our heads, we are subconsciously influencing ourselves to gobble every bite. Pay attention. By recognizing this you can make the choice to split an entrée or only eat an appetizer and a salad.

It's not cool to overeat. It's not funny, cute, or special. You don't have to eat what your friend or what your spouse eats. Choose to balance your hunger.

The path to health is moderation: calm, even and balanced. Do not be tempted by what everyone else does. Make your own mindful choices and be a positive influence for others. We can change our eating culture one choice and action at a time. Large servings are your friend but only if you use it to share with others. We eat to live; we do not live to eat.

May 5th

I acknowledge that moderation is the key to eating and drinking well.

Everything is okay – *in moderation.* Highlight that last phrase; it is imperative to your health journey. It's the aftermath of finishing the family sized bag of chips on the couch where we feel bloated or nauseous. A handful of tortilla chips is okay every now and again, it's the growing of a habit of gnawing on the chips that become the problem. The same goes for a glass of wine. With a steak, that lone glass of red wine compliments the meal by bringing out certain flavors. It's the several glasses that swerve you off track of your fitness goals.

Today, acknowledge that moderation is the key to eating and drinking well. You're allowed to indulge. That's what makes life so wonderful, the tiny luxuries that end the day on a high note. Simply don't make a habit out of the unhealthy choices. Make the unhealthier options only available for celebrations. Avoid turning your pantry into the chip aisle of the grocery store. Celebrate life with these treats. Find the balance in your journey.

May 6th

I have more energy and vitality when I eat well.

Your energy is fueled by a combination of the food you eat and how well your body processes it. This is a very close relationship. When you put nourishing and healthy foods in your body, you respond quicker to life more positively, and with increased clarity. Your body runs like a well-tuned engine.

When you eat high fat, high carb, or junk foods, your body likewise responds with dullness and slow motion. Test this out for a week. Don't concern yourself with weight. Pay more attention to how you feel. One meal at a time. You become energetic. Able to shift gears quickly. Without complaining. You turn eager and energetic.

You have more vitality when you eat well. Eat well today.

"A healthy outside starts from the inside." - Robert Urich

May 7th

I burst the myth that eating healthy is more expensive.

Eating healthy is not more expensive than eating poorly. I cringe when I hear this because I know the reality hasn't been put into perspective and people love an easy out. Here is what people don't want to know: the medical bills and doctor's visits considerably exceed what it costs to buy and eat healthier daily.

The $5 burger combo is cheaper per calories because it's calorie dense. Unhealthy and high in saturated fats, sodium, and sugar. 700 calories for $5? To leave you uncomfortable and overweight, that's not worth the money. That's 0.7 cents per calorie, but that same five-dollar bill could count for a 330-calorie salad.

Eating poorly on a regular basis will result in constant visits to the doctor. One doctor's bill averages $400, affecting your wallet, the healthcare system, and taxpayers. That's $6 per calorie for those monthly burgers. Don't even think about Emergency Room visits. Which lifestyle is cheaper? Invest in your health to invest in your life.

May 8th

I bring loving attention to my kidneys today.

Thank you, kidneys, for all you do. You strive hard every day by filtering waste from my blood. You regulate my blood pressure. You are indispensable to my health. My kidneys are under attack from unhealthy diets and harmful lifestyles, corrupting its proper functioning.

I am aware that my kidneys filter my blood and send toxins to my bladder, which are released during urination. I will bring loving attention to my kidneys by minimizing the toxins I put into my body, so my kidneys don't have to work tirelessly to fatigue or failure.

My dear kidneys, I will help you more and more by eating and drinking well. I will ease your job. I will pay attention to your health.

May 9th

I take time to enjoy the smell of food.

How wonderful is the smell of freshly baked bread? The coffee brewing in the early morning? The smell of turkey bacon as it sizzles? The feeling is enticing and comforting. This experience is not only reserved for slow mornings, you can access this feeling all the time. Activate your sense of smell by – you guessed it – smelling. Take precious time to observe the fragrance of the foods you eat.

Our noses and sense of smell are underutilized. When you practice smelling, an entirely new world opens for you to experience. We tend to let smells come to us and therefore they need to be strong for us to notice. We can open our awareness to follow the fragrances in the air and identify them.

Smell the rain, the fresh cut grass, or the toasty bonfire. Not just the perfume or your hand soap. Smell your food. Identify the flavors and enhance your eating experience. Smell. Then, eat.

May 10th

I am compassionate.

You have an untapped well source of compassion within you. Ask yourself, how have I shown compassion lately? Who have I been able to help through my resources or my kindness? Have I prayed for the wellbeing of anyone other than myself?

Whatever level of kindness you recognize in yourself is sufficient. Because wonderfully, each moment provides another opportunity to show some love. You can pray for someone's healing right now. You can contribute time or money to a cause. You can put a handwritten note or greeting card in the mail today.

What goes around comes around. Do unto others as you would have them do unto you. It's the law of attraction. Karma, if you will. When you are compassionate, you receive compassion and the world becomes a better place. Open the dam and release the river of compassion within you. Today.

May 11th

I will chew each bite of food 15-20 times.

We eat too fast. We chomp bites that are too big, sometimes unhooking our jaws. We chew three or four times and don't fully swallow what is in our mouth before we commit to the next bite. Have you been forced to rush through a meal before? It's animalistic. We force feed ourselves out of hunger and excitement. But in a mere matter of minutes, our entrees disappear. It's excessive and unnecessary for your body. Slow down. Make it easy for your organs to process the food. This is why you have indigestion problems, gas, or general discomfort in your gut. It's what you eat, yes, but it's also *how* you eat it.

When you slow down and chew, you taste your food. Savor it. Meals are meant to be enjoyed. The saliva in your mouth also helps to break down the food so your body can process it nicely. Then you're in store for a satisfyingly smooth move. Here's my advice on how to eat for your wellbeing. Take a small bite. Chew 15-20 times. Swallow. Do not take another bite before you swallow. Repeat. You'll eat less and digest more. Win-win.

May 12th

My daily affirmations keep me encouraged and able to achieve my goals.

Life can easily bring us down at times, but our default is designed for a life of happiness and abundance. Unfortunately, we've been conditioned to focus on the negative or always doing better, as if we are never good enough.

Here's good news for you-you are perfect just the way you are, right now. If you want to make changes to reach your God-given potential, shoot for the stars. Find your purpose. If you are changing to meet someone else's standards, then take stock and determine if it aligns with your true self.

Your daily affirmations keep you encouraged. They remind you of your awesome, unique, incredible self. The one that others might not see. The one you may be hiding. Affirmations remind you and encourage you to let your light shine for everyone. This is how you make the world a better place. By being you. Affirm your beauty daily. Thrive.

May 13th

I practice forgiveness.

It's been said that forgiveness is for you, not for the person you are forgiving. You need deep understanding and spiritual maturity to forgive someone who has betrayed you. Depending on how you were raised, forgiveness may not be an easy task. Start there.

Forgiveness is not so much for the wrong that was done, but rather an expression of understanding that this person is doing the best they can with the conditioning they have undergone. Much like you and I, we are the best we can be under our circumstances. Once we face these circumstances, we can change them.

Forgiveness will bring you peace. Practice on small things and large things always. The more you truly forgive, the more peace you will find.

"Forgiving what we cannot forget creates a new way to remember. We change the memory of our past into a hope for our future." - Lewis Smedes

May 14th

I spend more time outside with nature, which calms my mood and keeps my appetite satisfied.

Step outside. Take a breath. Breathe in through your nose, and out through your mouth, stretching your lips like a lion roaring to the sun. Focus on the way the light filters through the leaves on a tree, as the branches sway in the wind. Gaze at the bumblebee, which buzzes from one tulip to the next. Listen to the birds singing. Feel the blades of grass tickle your toes. Immerse yourself in the wonder that is nature. You are made up of the same cells and particles that make up the oak tree, the same organisms that allow the birds to soar, and the same water that nourishes the earth.

You *are* nature.

Choose to reflect on your connection to nature. Walk around the block to increase circulation. Breathe in the fresh air to rejuvenate the O^2 that enters each cell. Bask in the sunshine to take in some Vitamin D. Satisfy your craving for the ice cream sundae with the sweetness of nature. You'll feel relaxed, rejuvenated, and exceptional.

May 15th

I am aware that restaurants use techniques that cause weight gain.

Many restaurants focus on quantity and mass-production, where they tend to use techniques that promote weight gain. They pump saline water into meat to increase weight and shelf life of foods usability. You are left with aged food and a hefty amount of sodium without even knowing it.

The sugar, added fat, and salt ignites your taste buds. What follows is an addiction to certain flavors and their chemical reactions in your body. Not only that, but your meals are food dense with empty calories, no real nutritional value, and attributable to the building blocks for chronic illnesses.

Next time you dine at a restaurant, recognize these techniques. Ask your servers questions and make the best choices for you.

May 16th

I am healthy & vibrant.

We are what we believe. You must start seeing yourself now, the way you want to be in the future, and you will become that vision. Send that emotion of successful perfect health into your body right now and then go about achieving it. How, you ask?

Every successful person on earth first had to dream before they could do. They started out as hopeful beginners, and powered by desire. They followed a vision, plotted out the planning stages, and started working.

You are healthy and vibrant. Desire it with every cell in your body. Know it. Immerse yourself in the affirmation. Feel it where you already have perfect health and imagine it spreading to the rest of your body. You can create a wellbeing wildfire and catch your soul aflame. Let it spread to every corner of your life. How you think, what you eat, the environments you create and frequent. Clean the clutter of your home, smell the air during this springtime season, start fresh and a new every day, hour, and minute. You are healthy and vibrant.

May 17th

I recognize that I am influenced by my surroundings.

We travel from place to place during the routine of our day without noticing our surroundings. Yet, we are influenced by everything occurring around us. When we devote time to stillness and open our awareness, we compose the best choices for our lives.

When you wake up in the morning, admire your room in a new light. Observe the light complementing the walls and their color. What are you eating before you leave the house to face the outside world? What fuels you? What kind of company are you keeping at work? What group have you inadvertently joined?

Start from where you are. There is so much out there to take in and to give out. Put yourself in the best places for your wellbeing. Recognize.

May 18th

I make a conscious choice to avoid fatty foods.

There are good fats and bad fats. It's confusing to remember which is which so I'll keep it simple.

Liquid fats are better for health than solids. Vegetable oil is better than lard and most seed oils, like olive, are better than vegetable oil. Fried foods absorb and retain plenty of fat no matter the type of oil. Pan-fried is better than deep-fried. Sautéed, boiled, or baked is better than any kind of fried food for improving your health.

Make a conscious choice to avoid high-fat content. Choose the good fats in avocados and olive oil. Choose butter over the processed (and slightly mysterious) margarine. Choose ghee over butter. Many possibilities await you.

May 19th

I share my wellness affirmations with others who want encouragement.

Have you heard the saying "misery loves company"? It's inexplicably true. If you're in a negative space, you want others to join you in negativity. Shine a light on this perspective and turn the negative into positive, lasting relationships.

Choose the mindset to help and celebrate others' successes. When you can do this, it opens you up to achieve your own success. Attract positivity by supporting others positively. Which reminds me of another saying, "don't hate; appreciate." If someone has met a goal or lost more weight than you, give them a compliment. Set them as a role model. Feel good that if they can do it, so can you. Better still, when you make progress and see someone struggling or in doubt, encourage them. It's powerful. Share an affirmation or let them borrow the book. Improve your life by encouraging others.

May 20th

I am powerful.

You have the power to create the life you want. I understand this more and more every day, and you should, too. No one told me I was powerful until I reached a level in my career where my title presumed it. But, that's still not the power we're talking about here.

I had to learn my power on my own by observing my intentions and hitting a few tragedies. Tragedies, by the way, are powerful for awakenings, albeit extremely painful in their midst.

Wherever you are in your life right now, please know this - you are powerful beyond measure. You have the capability within you to do and accomplish whatever you want. Knowing this is crucial. It's a mighty step one in building the happy, healthy life you want. You are Powerful!

"Man is a universe within himself." – Bob Marley

May 21st

I recognize the emotional triggers that make me want to eat more.

Stress, boredom, sadness, and anger trigger our cravings, nudging us to the bag of buttery popcorn or box of frosted cupcakes. What do you bolt to after a hard workday, a breakup, or a loss? Cravings are memory based; you remember how your favorite fried chicken tasted during a somber mood, so you turn to those cravings to fill emotional turmoil. Sugars and salts release endorphins in the body, tricking you into fleeting happiness. Soon after, you're sucked into the couch, sluggish and bloated.

Be aware of what triggers you emotionally. Know your stressors or what makes you frown, so you can know what makes you smile. Increase your emotional intelligence to live consciously.

Today, realize your emotional relationship with food. I take note of how down emotions impact my progress. Refuse to fall victim to emotional cravings. Forbid angst or brooding to intercept your pathway of health. Instead, eat healthier so, in the future, you crave healthier options. With each juicy nectarine and crunchy carrot, your mood will boost. Fill your craving for positivity with positive choices.

May 22nd

I believe that God and those who love me accept me for who I am.

Higher power has many names. God, Allah, Yahweh, Brahman, to name a few. Maybe you have multiple gods. Maybe you're trying a couple on for size to see what fits you. More power to you (literally).

Whoever your higher power is, believe it accepts you for who you are. It and the universe's combined forces created you with each freckle, curve, and dimple pre-planned. This God loves you because it is you. You have pieces of stars and the universe planted in each pore.

The people who have your back, the ones who motivate you to join them in the gym and try the new juice bar on your block, also contain those star pieces. We all come from this universe and this higher power. Join forces with those who empower you. This spiritual support group love and accept you for who you are, through every gray hair and pimple.

Embrace the energy of the universe and the force of friendship. It will bring you to places you never thought you'd see.

May 23rd

I will release the past from my present.

Sometimes we're remarkably disappointed in ourselves where we drift into a funk. Instead of pushing past the ambiguous fog, we allow it to seep into whatever space is available, feeding into and intensifying our pessimism.

The last time I rummaged through my closet, I decided to slip on a pair of shorts, a pair that hid, hoping to one day be uncovered. As I dusted off these shorts, I was greeted not with a perfect fit, but to my dismay, they were too tight for public viewing. I raised my hands to the skies, shouting obscenities as I felt that ache of disappointment, creeping in slowly but surely.

I realized my energy immediately dropped. In an effort to regain my spirits, I threw on another pair of shorts. A comfortable pair - that fit. I looked fine. Even collected a couple compliments.

Today, I will release the past negative me and make positive choices in the present. I am eating well and reading my affirmations. I'll get reacquainted with those shorts another day.

"Only by acceptance of the past can you alter it."

-T.S. Elliott

May 24th

I am important.

You are vital to this world. Everything you do has an impact even more so than a butterfly fluttering its wings. Your thoughts have power. Your actions produce energy. Your energy attracts outcomes. Your outcomes design lives.

Stand up tall and look around you at this very moment. Say I am important. Feel the impact you have right now. Did you bring something to the space you are in? Have others noticed it? It's *you*. What energy are you bringing to the room? Is it joy, peace, intelligence or is it resentment and anger? You have the power to change the mood of places you go. The healthier and happier you are, the more good you do for the world.

You are vital to this world. You are so, so important.

My beliefs filter my experiences.

Your beliefs determine the lens with which you view the world. If you believe someone is untrustworthy, then you question and doubt everything they do. Those relationships lack trust and slowly deteriorate. Either adjust your belief or spend your time in trusting relationships.

If you believe someone is loyal and virtuous, you listen to that person and will follow them into difficult situations, like a soldier serving his commander or country. You always have choices, so it's important to examine your beliefs. Especially when you're in a negative headspace; things are usually not as bad as they seem.

Clean your lens. Remove the filters that block you from reality. It's like taking a picture out of focus or driving without your glasses.

Identify and experience your filter. Tint it to a rose color. Clear up the smudges to see the best and highest values you have. Then you'll see the best and highest in people. If their high is low, move on. But once you spritz those lenses of yours, you'll find there is goodness in everyone.

May 26th

I will walk today.

Walk today. Dedicate 15 minutes to simply walking. Even if you only walk to the corner and back today, mark that as a victory. Move. Small steps. Can't walk? Curl a can of soup for several reps. Lift your heaviest books. Find some mobility today outside of your norm.

We are a sedentary culture. We drive everywhere, sit and watch TV, and search the web. We end up psyching ourselves out as if we can't find the time to walk, so it's not worth doing anything. Rubbish. Anything is worth it. Everything is worth it. Start with a walk. Then, take it from there.

"Those who do not find time for exercise will have to find time for illness." –Edward Smith-Stanley

May 27th

I am successful.

What makes you successful? Success is whatever you define it to be. Start making more successes. Count the wins. Look for them. Create them. Celebrate them. You are successful. Create a goal and take small steps to achieve them. Then each step is a success. The world cannot make you feel small anymore. Only you can do that - and you won't.

Don't shrink away from your accomplishments. Feeling good about your achievements is a great thing to do. It is important even to draw in more and more positivity into your life. Ever heard the saying winners always win? Once you start seeing yourself as a winner, you become a winner. No need to brag or boast. Just be. Be the success you are. You are a winner.

"I find that the harder I work, the more luck I seem to have." – Thomas Jefferson

May 28th

I eat well because it gives me confidence.

There's a theory that to achieve the body of your dreams and to shed pounds, you should follow a regimen that concentrates 80% on diet and 20% on exercise. Eating well is crucial. Your body needs the vitamins, minerals, and electrolytes, which live in the lower half of the food pyramid. The better you eat, the better you feel.

How do you feel after you feast on the large meat-lover's pizza and six-pack of beer? But, how do you feel after a meal balanced with greens, carbs, and lean protein?

I eat well not because I want to lose weight, but because when I eat well, I am unstoppable. When I eat well, I am overcome with confidence. I feel divine, sublime, and captivating. Eating clean, beneficial food is a foolproof route to confidence. Eat for the confidence you desire when you ask out your crush, to walk into the boardroom, or for when you look in the mirror.

What gives you confidence? Find it. Harness it. Never let it go.

May 29th

I am my optimal state of wellbeing for me today.

Today, you are the healthiest you've ever been. You are the prime state of wellbeing for you. Not for your gym-nut neighbor or your lazy roommate, but for you.

Do the best you can each day. That's all you need to do. You don't need to be the best or start up a competition of wellness. Today, you are the healthiest you have been because each day you grow into a healthier being. Through the small steps and positive choices, you are developing a vision of health.

If wellbeing means you slept in an hour later than normal, then snooze the alarm. If health means you did a stretch session instead of cardio, then stretch it out. If wellness means you indulge in the *fettuccine alfredo*, then grab your fork and dig in.

You are the healthiest you've ever been not because of the scale, but through a combination of healthy choices, listening to your body and positive thinking. Be yourself and discover what makes you feel good. Then, find what makes you feel great.

May 30th

I eat food made from scratch.

Homemade food is the ultimate in good eating. Nothing compares for your overall wellbeing. The food is prepared from fresh ingredients with care to satisfy your taste buds. More often than not, the food is delicious and provides a feeling of satisfaction.

Mass-produced and processed foods are made with care for efficiency, low cost production, and increasing shareholder value. Your wellbeing and satisfaction are important in that it brings profit.

The good news is you have the power to choose what you eat. Choose foods made fresh and from scratch. Foods where someone put individual time and care into its production. The love and freshness combine to give you maximum results - health and wellbeing. Start from scratch and eat from scratch.

May 31ˢᵗ

I am in harmony.

Harmony is like a melody. Think of a song you like where the musical notes are just magical. Whenever it plays you feel a little pang in your heart. Or a singer who hits a note or has the vocals of an angel.

Life has a flow. A rhythm. We all take part in this cosmic dance, like waves in an ocean. If you are still enough, you can feel your place within it; like a perfectly placed note in a song or the cherry on top of your ice cream sundae.

You must move, bend, flex, and flow to find your place in the world. You can lead or follow. Be like the wind, fire, earth, or water.

Or, simply, what do you feel best doing? When do you feel most alive and apart of this flow? I notice when I'm connecting with others; I like to get things done and I love to laugh. When I perform these acts at once, I am in true harmony.

What are your ingredients? What notes make your melody? You were created to be in harmony. It's time to find your flow.

Summer.

June 1st

Gratitude + Forgiveness = Love.

There are countless ways to define love. One way to think of it is through gratitude and forgiveness.

I think of love as accepting others no matter their personality or choices. It's knowing they might fault or fail, but supporting them anyway. Forgiveness is a strength, not many possess. But if you can forgive your loved ones, you grasp a power within yourself.

Being grateful for the people who inspire you, who make you laugh, even the ones who show tough love – all these colorful personalities and shining faces create a hub of happiness. You are home when you are with these people because you love them. You are grateful for your relationships because they'll always forgive you and you'll always forgive them.

Self-love works similarly. To love yourself, forgive yourself for past wrongdoings. To love yourself, be grateful for your life. You are unique. You are different. Give thanks for your individuality. You find gratitude through forgiveness and forgiveness through gratitude. And it always equals out to love.

June 2nd

I am reinventing myself into the person I always wanted to be.

It's enchanting when you realize you are your own creator on this earth. Who do you want to be? By following these daily affirmations, you've decided to have a happier life centered around your total wellbeing. You have infinite possibilities to create the new you. When you change your eating, you change your body chemistry. When you change your thinking, you redevelop your brain's neural pathways. You literally become a new you.

When I quit the corporate world, a good friend treated me to a *beverage* on my last day to celebrate. On that Friday afternoon, we sat outside in the June sun. I lifted my head up towards the sky and inhaled a deep breath. Out of nowhere, a tear rolled down my face. She was worried. "Are you okay?" I assured her I was and claimed, "I'm finally the person I always wanted to be."

Be you today. And every day.

June 3rd

I am blessed with a new vision for my life.

I recently read something that people don't change much after their 30's. They settle into conformity. Ride out raising the kids, followed by looking at retirement plans, and before you know it, you're setting your affairs in order. Oh, and don't forget to throw in a mid-life crisis somewhere to shake things up.

In that sense, I'm not mad at mid-life crises. More and more people are living to be 100. Why would I want to have all the best, exciting times of life for the first 30 years and spend the next 70 in a holding pattern? Passively watching your life elapse, like a plane circling the airport waiting to land. No way. Not for me, and not for you.

Create a vision for your life. Extend it through an entire lifetime. Make sure you have the vitality and energy to live your interesting and meaningful life. You do this by including your wellbeing and health in your vision. You are blessed. Vision your new healthy life and then go live it.

June 4th

In every moment, I can choose from infinite possibilities.

You can choose to read this passage. Skip through the book. Throw it in the trash. Give it away. Close it. Destroy it with dog-eared pages. Read it from cover to cover. There are a million things you can do right now just with this book alone.

As you go along today, realize that with every step, action, & breath, you have an infinite number of choices you can make that impact your health, your life, and the lives of those around you. You can go right or left. Have breakfast or not. Coffee or tea. Orange Juice or make it a mimosa. Call off sick. Put in overtime to wow them with that presentation. The list goes on. Do what you want. Be what you need.

Pay attention. You choose your life with every choice. Choose wisely. Choose mindfully. Choose your health.

You have infinite possibilities.

June 5th

I bring loving attention to my liver today.

God bless my liver. I have done a number on it over the years. With no regard for my liver, I have consumed many substances and foods that are difficult to process and work directly against my wellbeing. But my liver, the overachiever it is, keeps on working. Harder and harder. Faithfully. Relentlessly. My liver is like a troop in the armed forces. My liver is a Green Beret; exhaustive training, fighting battles, and often times in cover operations on enemy soil.

Be kind to your liver. You only have one and it truly is one of the hardest working, resilient, and underappreciated organs in your body. Everyone talks about the heart, lungs, and kidney. The liver, though always last, is the largest internal organ.

Place your hand on the upper right position of your abdomen and say, "Liver, I salute you!"

June 6th

I overcome the struggles of my health journey by helping others.

Sometimes distancing yourself from your troubling situations allows you to find the solution. The same goes for this health journey. Maybe you need to clear your head with a walk outside or a talk with a friend. I find one of the most rewarding and memorable ways to overcome the struggles of this health journey is through helping others.

One of my favorite ways to do so is through food sharing. It's a way to help others while helping yourself. With food sharing, you cut back on food waste, miniaturize your portions, and develop supportive relationships with those who are on this journey, too. When you share, you don't overeat or overindulge. When you share food, you share light, happiness, and positivity.

Maybe someone couldn't afford groceries this week or also wants to cut back on portion size. Team up with your friends, neighbors, or those in your community. The *UGottaEat* app can help you reach out to others and find people who want to share. When we help others, we help ourselves. Through compassion for others, you find compassion for yourself.

June 7th

I am thankful for the weather today.

Everyone has a weather condition that they live with every day. Every single one of us has that in common. It may be sunny, rainy, snowy, or just gray. No matter what your conditions, take a minute to be thankful.

Recognize that the sun must shine to give energy. The rain must come and water the green earth so we can eat and see the beauty of flowers. The winter must come to shed the old so we can be refreshed by the renewing of spring.

Everything in life has a cycle of outcomes. Try not to look at them as negative or positive, but as the conditions that sustain us. That allows our food to grow. That nourishes our bodies and gives life to our loved ones. Today and every day, start by giving thanks for the weather; Mother Nature can feel underappreciated, too.

"Nature is the art of God." – Dante Alighieri

June 8th

I read books and magazines that promote health.

You become what you think about. What you feed your mind becomes what you feed your body. Junk television and junk food have the infamous pairing of peanut butter and jelly. Expand your mind with reading materials that instill motives around your search for wellbeing. Subscribe to a wellness magazine. *Fitness. Prevention. Men's Health* and *Women's Health. Runners World. Yoga.* There's a magazine for every health interest, so narrow down yours. Or treat yourself – buy the whole magazine shelf. Buy a book that informs you on the latest and greatest in the wellness world, one that is motivational and inspirational as much as it is educational. An autobiography of an athlete or ballerina maybe. Think outside of your normal reading material.

The things you keep your mind on educate you and influence your day-to-day decisions. Knowledge is power. Listen to a podcast. Watch a documentary once a month. Join a running group. Become a part of a community that advocates for the type of lifestyle and body choice you desire. Either it will bring you along, or you will bring someone else along, to wellness.

June 9th

I am excited!

Stand up. Right now! Raise your energy. Electrify each action and movement. Tackle a goal with zeal and gusto. Shout to the rooftops. Find at least one aspect of this diet and wellness journey that excites you and start the positive motion in your life. One lively example can deliver you the energy needed to raise your vibration and prompt joy. Your energy matters.

Transform your look. Dabble in a hobby. De-clutter your closet. Volunteer at a food bank. Call all your friends to catch up with; dial-up those with names that start with the letter Z and work your way to A. Whatever you want. Change and action, no matter how small, will help motivate you to do and accomplish everything and anything.

You need energy. Everything is made up of energy. Harness it. Don't overlook it. Use it. Do it. Jump up and down. Look at baby pictures. Dance until you break a sweat. Anything. Just get excited. A journey begins with a single step.

"I am seeking. I am striving. I am in it with all my heart." – Vincent van Gogh

June 10th

I am thankful for my local grocer.

Where do you get your food? Probably from a grocery store or a supermarket. If you're really lucky, you're even growing and farming some of your produce. Suffice it to say, your grocery store is probably within a 5-10-mile radius of your house.

Give a special bit of time to recognize where your food is birthed and its growth. The grocery or market has taken the time to build an infrastructure to make foods available for you to eat. We sometimes become cynical and think they only do it for the money. To be clear, there are much easier and higher margin careers to pursue for the money. I'm not certain your local grocer is in it for the quick cash.

Most grocers start with a desire to provide good food. The more local the market, the better. Local markets are continuously promoting sustainability, organics, and wellness. They support your local economy. They care. Send a thankful blessing to your local grocer.

June 11th

I eat fast food strategically.

___

Fast food and fast casual dining have overrun many communities. These restaurants offer large or value sized servings quickly. Lickety-Split. With our busy culture, the convenience appeals to many.

Since you're focusing on eating for wellbeing, you can choose wisely when to eat fast food. Recognize that the portions are immense. The food is mass-produced for commerciality. Additional fat, sugar, and preservatives are added. Calories are doubled from the same item cooked at home. Be smart and aim for the options that don't scream "heart attack" or "diabetes." Some of these fast food options offer calorie counts. Use them to increase your awareness of the meal itself.

Be strategic. When I'm in a pinch, I throw a couple pieces of fruit and granola bars in my bag. When I'm in a situation where friends are serving grilled burgers at the seasonal cookout or when relatives bring fried options to the family reunion, I partake out of respect (but also because they add that secret ingredient called "love"). I keep my eyes open, take the hit, and keep moving in the right direction for my overall strategy of wellbeing.

June 12th

I walk 30 minutes daily.

Activity is important. It's essential to your wellbeing; cardio is a common prescription from doctors, fitness enthusiasts, and health coaches everywhere to reduce your risk of disease. It helps to lose weight, strengthen the heart muscle, and improve blood flow. If your body is moving and flowing, you can almost feel it in your bloodstream. Tiny little blood cells dancing through the corridors of your veins, looking good and feeling better.

The simplest of all activity which most of us are blessed with is the ability to walk. A brief walk of 30 minutes per day will slowly activate groundbreaking improvements. Not once per week, but consistently. Shoot for every day but make three days a week your minimum; if you average five days a week, you're on a roll. Walk briskly along a leveled road. Hike a steep hilltop. Don't stroll. Work up a small but mighty sweat. Walking is an exercise, and it's an exercise to strengthen your most crucial muscle - your heart.

It can be tricky to find the time but decide to make the time. Split up the 30 minutes into intervals. Take advantage of your work breaks. Improve your life with simple things. Walk.

June 13th

Today I bless my arms.

Thank you, arms, for navigating the details of each movement I make. You give the warmest hugs and shake the strongest hands. You allow my hands to reach, granting me the ability to push and pull, lift and lower.

Because of you, I can hold things, move things, and even decorate you with adornments or jewelry. I maneuver vehicles, write out love notes, type up projects, and play games with my arms. You're a good friend to me.

I will strengthen you through more exercises. I will eat well to keep you lean and vibrant. I will love more so you can keep giving those great hugs.

Thank you, arms. I will treat you well.

June 14th

It is my intention to have an alert mind.

The mind clouds itself every now and again, a haze casting itself onto your memory. You may forget what you are saying mid-sentence. You could walk upstairs and forget what you meant to grab. You might leave your wallet at the grocery store. This occurs more as you age, but you can slow this phenomenon.

I think of the mind-body connection as a screen door, a kitchen colander, or a lint catcher in the dryer. When there is lint or debris clogging the holes, the air or liquid flow is blocked or slowed. When you rid your lint catcher of its dust, you reveal a clear and clean screen, ready to take on another day's challenges, wool sweaters and all.

Similarly, eating well will detox your body and liberate the layers of film and buildup out of your body so you function at your highest energy and clarity. Add the intentionality of presence and awareness, and you will improve your quality & quickness with amazing speed. Set intentions to pay attention. Wake up. There's a whole day ahead of you. Make it count.

June 15th

I check social media after I eat.

Social media is as entertaining as watching a movie; there's action, comedy, drama, and romance. You scroll through the events of other people's lives, clicking on profiles to catch up on old acquaintances or a past event. Sit in on a live taping of a graduation or a protest captured by someone in attendance. It's like a tunnel - you continuously progress deeper until you're burrowed in (or come up for air to post your own incredible life stories).

It is impossible for your food to compete with the focus of your phone. And trust me, your food is way more important to your wellbeing than who liked your post or the hourly updates of the friend from high school. If they are that important, you would communicate with them directly.

Everyone else can wait until after you eat. Give your full awareness to your priority of wellbeing. Direct your focus to what matters to your mind, body, and spirit. When you eat, *eat*.

June 16th

I am empowered.

How do you feel, right now, in this moment? Are you sleepy? Are you wide-awake? Are you bored, lonely, or sad? What about alive and curious? What if I told you that you are powerful? How would you feel then?

You *are* powerful. Say to yourself aloud, "I am empowered." Put that superhero soundtrack on your stereo and feel the wind at your back. Imagine standing atop a building with your hands on your hips and your chin held high.

Whether you have a monogrammed initial on your chest or simply, the shirt your wearing, know that you are empowered through each positive decision you make. You are empowered because you make a promise to better yourself each day. You are empowered with each exercise video and hefty salad. You become stronger and more confident through your healthy choices. And when you're confident in your choices, you find confidence in yourself.

You aren't any old boring sidekick - you are the main event. You are powerful. Now go save the city (or continue eating your vegetables, whatever works).

June 17th

I ask my higher power to order my steps.

Always remember you are not alone. Too often, we fatigue ourselves attempting to understand the confusions of life or struggle to accomplish a goal with our own power and might. Today, remember there are forces that help govern your life that you can lean on, universal energies that support you during both the marvelous moments and the troublesome.

Your health and wellbeing is a direct result of your actions and choices. Today, choose to lean on your higher power. Think beyond your five senses. Consider the universe's plan for you. Instead of losing your temper or succumbing to doubt or sadness, be quiet and still throughout the day. Meditate. Listen to your intuition. Pay attention to that gut feeling. Notice the *déjà vu*. Coincidences are not accidents or crazy chance - it's the universe talking to you.

Choose to listen and receive the messages. Take action for your best life now. The universe delivers happiness to everyone. Listen, and you'll hear how.

"God is our refuge and strength, a very present help in times of trouble." – Psalms 46:1

I stay hydrated.

Invest in a high quality water bottle. Hydration keeps the supply of oxygen and blood flowing through your body. It prevents headaches and delivers the nutrients from your diet throughout your body, providing energy with each sip. Supermodels and professional athletes everywhere accredit hydration to their success, so something must be working.

Keep a bottle of water with you always. Splurge on the eco-friendly reusable types that withstand your busy lifestyle. Fill it to the brim whenever you can. If your bottle is 16 ounces, drink four bottles a day. Witness the changes in your body from simply drinking more water. You think clearer and move more swiftly. Hydration reveals plump skin, shiny hair, and a thin waist. The more water you drink, you tend to eat smaller portions, so gulp down a glass before a meal. If you think it's too bland, squeeze fresh lemon or muddle some cucumbers into it. Soak fruit in a water bottle overnight and sip throughout the day.

Stay hydrated today; I can't think of a reason why you shouldn't.

June 19th

I am imagining my healthier body in the future.

It is important to set goals. These are intentions to where we hope to arrive to; they are destinations on a map. We make specific goals and throw numbers & data in like salt and pepper. "I want to lose 20 pounds" or "I need to fit into a size 8" or my favorite, "If I only eat 500 calories for lunch that means I can have pizza for dinner."

We can be just as impactful, if not more, by envisioning ourselves as we want to be. Thoughts lead to words, and words lead to action. Focus on the thoughts. Cultivate positive intentions and water your garden of goals. See yourself the way you want to be. Each day you will near that vision through your words and actions. It is important to start with the end in mind. See it. Know it's possible. Feel the emotion of contentment swirl in your body like a hurricane when you achieve your ideal health. Call up this vision and this feeling when you are choosing between wellbeing and temporary taste. It will remind you that health feels better than food tastes. We're in it for the long haul, gang.

I am unapologetically me.

You are wildly unique. There is no one on this earth like you. You don't share the same thoughts, aspirations, or talents with anyone. No one can tell a story like you, or sing like you, or has that infectious laugh of yours.

Today, the media repeatedly shows us images and videos of what we should be doing, how we should act, and who we should be. But you don't need that negative energy. You don't have time for those who don't support you. And if you want to change, change not for the media, but for you.

You thrive on this magnificent journey. You better yourself every day with each step and balanced meal. Your spinach salad lunch is rearing you up for your big solo. You prevail as a rock star and the stadium is filled with glow-sticks of adoration. Fans are lining up backstage just to peek a glimpse at you. If you walked into your dressing room, you'd see hundreds of roses.

I am unapologetically me. Be unapologetically you.

June 21st

I eat fruit as a snack today.

I'm working on the discipline to snack mindfully throughout the day. Some amazing people don't snack at all. Others need chips or a scoop of ice cream between each meal. What makes us all so different? Our choices.

We are all born with certain traits and become conditioned by our environment & surroundings. Ultimately, however, our choices are ours to make. Snacking is often an overlooked culprit in our journey to wellness. Focus on your typical snack. Is it a donut or a candy bar? Or do you keep three pieces of fruit on your desk? Do you grab handfuls of candy or mints from co-worker's community bowls?

Today, focus on eating healthy fruits and veggies as snacks. Or skip the snack if you can. Snack wisely.

June 22nd

I am living in the present moment.

Accept yourself right now for who you are. Accept how you look, your hair, and the color of your skin. Accept your level of education, your relationships, and your job. In this present moment, accept yourself and your external station in life.

Now, delve deeper and accept who you *really* are right now. Accept your heart and the love you feel for others. Accept how you show compassion & care for your family. Accept how much you matter in this world to your family, your home, your plants, your pets. Accept that you are a part of this world and therefore the world is also a part of you.

In this moment, you are. No need to worry about the past or fret about the future. Be your best and highest self. Now. Make the best choices in this moment. Do it again, and the next moment. No need for regrets because each moment is fresh. Your wellbeing is improving now. Be present.

June 23rd

I am optimistic.

Live life through a lens of positivity and it will open you up to successfully achieving your goals and happiness. Society, parents, colleagues, and friends teach us that worry, expecting the worse, and having a plan B (and C and D) is the way to success. They mean well and carry good intentions, attempting to navigate us through life with practical considerations. However, worry and angst do not equal success.

If you aspire true happiness and abundance, you must see it and believe it. You can't know you are going to achieve your goals *and* be worried about failure at the same time. Notice when you say something positive who and how many times people will say, "yes… but," and proceed to list the possible downsides. Only listen for the positives. Breakthrough the barriers of negative thinking. Be the successful minority.

Play to your strength. Your strength is your optimism. Your ability to live in the light of life's situations, not the darkest. Believe.

"Choose to be optimistic, it feels better." – Dalai Lama

June 24th

I park a conscious distance away so I can walk more.

Parking lots exasperate me. Like mice in a maze, we crawl around dozens of rows to find the perfect spot. And for what?

Today, park further away. Meet your step quota. If you're lucky enough to own a device to inform you of your step count, use it diligently. Your body is not meant to sit at a desk day in and day out, only to move to the couch when you return home. Walk when you need to walk. Stretch when you need to stretch. Move because you need to move.

Parking a conscious distance away is a simple solution to increasing your daily movement. Find other ways you can walk more. Walk up the stairs an extra flight or two. Step outside and tour the neighborhood. It's small steps like these that can make the greatest difference.

June 25th

I focus on my wellbeing.

Whatever you devote your attention to will thrive. Think back over your life and the events that stand out will be the ones that you gave effort and attention. Good or bad, the things you give attention to will manifest in your life.

When you focus on relationships, they take center stage whether you were engaged to be married, trying online dating, or fighting with your best friend. Allow your wellbeing to step under the spotlight. Light up the stage and start a new period in your life of focusing on your wellbeing. Focus on eating foods that impart a healthy, sensational feeling, not ones that leave an "I'll start over again tomorrow" reaction. Focus on rest for energy and on positive, creative environments.

Focus and be well.

June 26th

I am pleased with my looks.

Find three things about your appearance that you like. Do it right now. List them here. Don't overthink it. You can make a new list every day. Is it your nails? Complexion? That you have your mother's eyes? Healthy hair? Express gratitude to your body and it will express gratitude back to you by radiating health and happiness.

Stop saying the infamous lines leading to the rabbit hole of low self-esteem – "I'm fat." "My waist is gone." "I hate my double chin."

Negativity breeds negativity.

It amazes me how often in a day I hear people say negative things about themselves that they would never allow others to say to their loved ones. You are your most precious loved one; you are your best friend.

Speak positively to yourself. Focus on what you are pleased about and then eventually you will be pleased with your entire self. You are worthy. You are enough. You are perfect the way you are. Start seeing yourself the way I see you. The way the universe made you.

"Love yourself first, and everything else falls into line."
– Lucille Ball

June 27th

I am changing the weekend habit to over-indulge.

We work diligently during the week to the extent where each weekend has transformed into a recurring holiday. We develop the habit of celebrating with food and drink, and it becomes our weekend ritual with our closest acquaintances. Happy Hour Friday after work drinks with your co-workers, Saturday barbecues on a sunny afternoon of grilling out, Sunday family dinners. The social interaction is needed and comforting. It lowers your stress levels to burn off steam. No wonder we look forward to the weekend – it's filled with the makings of marvelous memories.

The only issue I see is the over-consumption. Do we need the extra beer at Happy Hour? Can we abstain from the wide variety of junk foods at the cookout?

We *can* socialize without mind-altering drinks and heavy-laden foods. Don't fall victim to the same old routine. Mix up your days – visit a museum with friends, hit the beach with family, or start a book club with your bookworm coworkers. Use the weekend to focus more on the relationships and not the food.

June 28th

I recognize that alcohol slows my metabolism.

Metabolism is a trickster. First it eludes you, appearing as a subtle side effect; but next, it shows up on your scale. Why isn't everybody talking about this? We need to increase our awareness about metabolism, like flu shots in the fall and allergies in the spring.

It is important that you understand it. Not only does your metabolism slow with each passing day, alcohol progressively slows it down. So if you are aging (as we all do every single second), and want to have optimal health and vitality, alcohol is an extra weight dragging down your goal.

Recognizing this, drink moderately. Put your exercise and positive eating habits in overdrive to compensate for the lack of burn from drinking. Or, don't drink. You choose, but choose with your eyes wide open to reality.

June 29th

My positive choices create a chain reaction toward my goals.

There are universal laws revealed by Isaac Newton, a 17th-century scientist, on the laws of motion. The first law, the Law of Inertia, concludes that an object at rest stays at rest, and an object in motion stays in motion with the same speed and in the same direction unless acted upon by an unbalanced force.

Basically - objects keep on doing what they are doing. When you make positive choices consciously, you continue to build upon your successes. Ever wonder why the rich become richer, or some have a perpetual lucky streak? They found their starting points and stayed in motion toward their goal.

This law works for you, too. The interruption is the resistance. The clause is known as "acted upon by an unbalanced force" provokes negative thinking, toxic relationships, and bad influences. Make positive choices one by one and eliminate those unbalanced forces that try to slow you down.

June 30th

Today I honor my body as a temple.

Your body houses your soul. Your body houses your heart, which loves. And it houses your mind, which thinks for you. Your body is a temple. A precious container that keeps and holds all your most valuable treasures... What do you treasure? Your jewelry? Maybe it's in a jewelry box. Your car? Probably wish you had a garage for that. Your clothes? There are businesses now dedicated to building fantastical closets.

We devote time throughout our days to honor these "containers." And still, we take our bodies for granted. Your body is magnificent. Doctors and scientists still don't truly understand how it works. The brain is a complete mystery and it's a journey to find cures for what ails you. If we honor our bodies as the most precious container we have, we enjoy health & happiness. We won't need to know all the mechanics because she's purring like a kitten and all is well.

"Do you know that your bodies are temples of the Holy Spirit, who is in you, whom you have received from God? You are your own; you were bought at a price." - 1 Corinthians 6:19-20

July 1st

I have courage.

My daughter was about to pledge a sorority and she confided in me that she was afraid. I heard this 25 years before from one of my own sisters as we entered the pledge process. My response hadn't changed - "you're supposed to be scared."

You cannot show your courage, confront a foe with all your strength, or stand up for a cause unless there is something to push against. A resistance. A barrier. A challenge. Be grateful for the chance to show your courage, have the ability to win a victory, or overcome a defeat (and what joy there is in it for you, the overcomer). Without the ebb & flow, everything is flat. There's a time for a still sea, but there are also times for big waves. Go surfing. Crash into the water. Ride the wave.

It's difficult making healthy choices, like going to a work dinner and not taking advantage of the free steak, flowing drinks, or complimentary dessert. But it's *supposed* to be difficult.

Anything worth having is worth working for. You are worth it. Be courageous.

July 2nd

I eat only one dessert this week.

Having a sweet tooth is not an excuse to purchase a sheet of brownies or a family-sized pint of the double-chocolate chunk.

This week, eat only one dessert. Donate the sugar cookies and give your homemade muffins to your neighbor. You don't need a daily dose of sugar. Usually, you are ingesting sugar from unsuspecting places, like your fruit and yogurt parfait or your coffee creamer. Having sugar every night or even every other night creates a habit. Soon, you become addicted to the substance, sniffing it out at convenience store aisles.

Save dessert for one day this week. Plan it out ahead of time so you have a set date and don't veer off track. Reserve dessert for those special nights, whether it's the weekly meet up with friends or date night with your partner. Dessert isn't meant to be mundane or ordinary but is baked and crafted as a celebration. When you dedicate one day to dessert, it makes that dessert better. The taste is rich and the colors are bold. You remember how great it tastes. It becomes a sensory experience, rather than a daily duty. Regain that experience by allotting one special night this week for that hand-crafted gelato. Your taste buds will thank you.

July 3rd

I connect with people who improve and motivate me.

I once received tickets from a dear friend for a prestigious literary awards ceremony. It was scheduled for a weeknight, the weather was rainy, and I was confronted with the struggle of what to wear - clearly these are reasons to scrap the awards for a night on the couch.

Deeper than the environment around me, I held a curiosity about these authors. What had they written? What kind of organization is presenting the awards? What topics (and who) are important to our culture?

I imagined I might meet some famous authors. I might learn what it takes to succeed. I might be motivated by the books themselves. They must be noteworthy or at least decent; obviously, there's an entire ceremony around their accomplishments. At a minimum, I would be enveloped in the energy and company of people who inspire. I adore literature and interesting topics. Thus, I attended, despite the rain or the last minute outfit decision. I went. I am motivated. I win!

Who motivates you?

July 4th

I acknowledge we are all connected.

Scientists theorize living creatures descended from the stars. The atoms and elements, which allow the stars to shine in the night sky, live within our skin. We are sprinkled with remnants of the cosmos, pieces of planets, and the intricate secrets of stardust.

Honor the magic of the universe within yourself and others. Each human being, animal, plant, and microscopic organism originated from the same explosion. We all have hearts that beat, lungs to breathe, and a soul that glows - we are all connected. Regardless of gender, ethnicity, sexuality, or social status, we are all here on this earth together. Acknowledge this grand connection. Know that with each sentence interruption, each late arrival, or each smile, your actions will affect someone else.

Spread kindness today. Know that we all inhabit this planet together. Work with one another. Encourage and motivate each other. Together, let's rebuild what it means to be healthy. Let's develop an overall wellbeing that will transcend space and time. With each smile, let's add to the universe. Together.

July 5th

I change my body, by changing how I think about my body.

Too often we are too hard on ourselves. We criticize our stomachs, arms, and backs. We dream of slim waistlines and toned thighs. Our ankles are swollen, knees bruised, and our cheeks don't shine like it used to.

Today, I will focus on the awesome things my body does for me. I can taste wonderful flavors, see beautiful sights and art, touch soft pillows, hear music that makes me move, and smell aromas that bring back memories of my childhood.

Thank you, legs and ankles, for taking me where I need to go.

Thank you, arms and hands, for your reach and your grasp.

Thank you, breasts, for feeding my children.

Thank you, stomach, for digesting and holding so much together.

Thank you, organs, for all you do (that I don't even understand).

Thank you, mind, for choosing gratitude and to think positively about my body.

July 6th

It is my intention to serve.

Focusing on problems sometimes makes it harder to get out of your own way. You attract what you focus on. It's a small but extremely important nuance. Focus on the solutions to find a solution. Focus on the problem, and you will add to the problem.

If you set an intention to serve, it is this mechanism that allows you to change that focus to the positive. Serving means to help or be of use. When you are in a helpful mode, whether to others or to yourself, you create a more powerful mindset that clarifies the solutions. Gain a sense of clarity by serving your needs and the needs of others. Sometimes focusing on topics besides your problems can grant you the clarity to a solution. It's a change of scenery that opens your mind, like a breath of fresh air.

Serve yourself today. Embrace fresh food. Serve a friend and bring them something delicious and healthy. Intend to serve.

July 7th

I drink non-alcoholic beverages today.

How does alcohol affect your daily routine? Are you more willing skip those daily chores? Now, think about how a day when you don't drink differs. You probably complete your to-do list with the gusto of an intern hoping to impress. You might think of some creative ideas for your next business venture.

Happy hour or weekend specials don't mean you need to throw away your productivity with a trip to the brewery. And the unfortunate result of drinking is unhealthy decisions for food. You aren't interested in the kale, but instead, order the deluxe pizza for one.

Today, drink non-alcoholic beverages. Clear your mind through water, tea, and fresh fruit juice. Notice how clear your day or evening becomes. Notice how hydrated you feel when you wake up the next morning.

July 8th

I am being kind to myself.

What is the most loving thing you can do for yourself? Today, sprinkle these little moments of happiness into your daily living. You don't have to wait for a spa day or a birthday. Gift yourself small, random acts of kindness. Put on your favorite sweats and snuggle on the couch. Watch a drama or an action movie alone. Put on your best ensemble for no reason. Who is to say you can't look incredible today? You are obliged to this life because it's *your* life.

Flip through an old photo album. Take a nap. Sit outside in the sun. Listen to the rain as it hits your window. Play with your dog. Amuse yourself and take a romantic date alone. Put fresh flowers in the house. Spray on a touch of perfume or cologne. Give yourself an honest compliment and accept it graciously. This is you. Build yourself up to where you rightfully belong: healthy & happy.

Stop the self-criticism and enjoy yourself today. Practice loving the reflection in the mirror. Be kind to you.

"No one can make you feel inferior without your consent." – Eleanor Roosevelt

July 9th

My thoughts choose what I will eat today.

When you think about food, what are you thinking about? If you don't know what you're going to eat this week, or even today, you are leaving your health to chance. Don't leave it to chance. Pause and take time to decide how and what you will eat this week.

Make a grocery list. Plan to eat entrée salads or lean fish at the work dinners. Think about how to keep healthy snacks handy. If you've made plans to visit an amusement park, you can assume there is nothing healthy there. So, think about eating before and what you will eat after. Throw an apple in your backpack for while you're there.

And so be it, if you choose to treat yourself to those wonderful funnel cakes or elephant ears, where powder sugar falls gracefully slow. At least you made a conscious choice. Your thoughts are in control, not the marketplace.

I choose lightness and laughter.

Give yourself a break. Take it easy. Be intentional about your light; take that tiny flicker and add more fuel to the fire. Bring levity, brilliance, starbursts, lyrical harmony, dance, and creativity to the present moment.

We focus on our burdens and stresses - bills, careers, and failed relationships dominate our attention to where we forget the little sparks of happiness that pop up throughout our days.

Give yourself a mental vacation. Find the joy in small surprises. Happily, ignore those who are filled with hate. Dedicate tomorrow to your responsibilities and take today for yourself to find the light in your life.

Watch a comedy, call your funniest friend, and eat something that won't leave you bloated and sleepy. Get a smoothie. If you're feeling crazy, top it off with some chocolate. Just enjoy life today. Then, every day.

"Enjoy yourself, enjoy yourself, enjoy yourself with me." –Michael Jackson

July 11th

I am able to break old habits and create new ones.

Habits do not have a hold on you. They may grasp your attention for a while, but once you recognize that you can change them, you have control. Habits are breakable and changeable. They do not have to live forever unless you choose.

Habits are like a houseplant. If it's a good habit, like exercising and eating right, you water it a little each day. Don't overdo the watering can or try to feed it. It will die.

You can create powerful new habits. You don't have to quit your sugar addiction cold turkey. Start with one step. Just one.

Today, you have the power to skip the caffeine. Avoid the donut shop. Say your affirmations daily. Spend time outside, with your loved ones, and with yourself. You choose. You own your habits. Both old and new.

July 12th

I perform at peak condition.

Check in with your body to make sure you know your peak condition. Liken it to having your car serviced. The brakes are checked, oil changed, and air-filled tires. When everything is checked and serviced, you have a smooth ride. Your body is like this. Give yourself a 5-point tune up. Are you in 5-star condition?

1. Morning Energy – Do you wake up tired or excited to face the day?

2. Skin and Eyes – Are you blotchy with acne or smooth & supple? Are my eyes bright or red with circles?

3. Digestion – Am I bloated or happy, with all my parts running smoothly?

4. Pain-Free – Scan your body from head to toe. Headaches, pressure points, joint pain? Or loose and easy?

5. Clarity – Is my mind clear and focused? Or am I foggy, forgetful, and weighed down by negative emotions?

Rate yourself. Are you in 5 star condition? Hitting on all cylinders? You can be. Food is medicine. Write your prescription today.

July 13th

Today I bless my butt.

If there's "butt" in the affirmation, you can bet it'll be a good one. I have had a love-hate relationship with my butt my whole life until I became mindful. It's too big, too flat, or too lumpy - actually, it's perfect.

Songs have been written about the rear-end, the booty, the derriere, the tush, the bum. It's been given several nicknames based on its popularity. The *gluteus maximus* muscles keep us moving and strong. They provide a foundation for our movement and relaxation.

Today, send blessings to your butt. Thank it for powering your legs, for communing with your hips, and for always finding a place to sit. Forgive me, butt, for my past complaining and recognize that I, and others, appreciate you.

July 14th

I am at my perfect weight.

Determine in your spirit where you want to be and visualize it. Declare it. What does it look like? Or better yet, what does it feel like? This is where you are to spend your mental energy as you travel this journey to wellbeing - with your emotions. Your feelings and intuition are accurate guides, much more so than your 5 senses.

Start with your why. Why do you want to be a certain weight? If it's only to fit in a certain outfit or to look like you did when you were younger, that motivation will evade your goal. It's surface and will produce shallow results. You may reach your weight through sheer might, but you won't be able to stay there.

Your why must align with your spirit. With your best and highest values and qualities. Vanity is not it. Health & happiness, energy & vitality, or love & joy will get you there. Feel your perfect weight. State your why. Meet me at the finish line.

July 15th

Today I send silent blessings to those who struggle with their body image, for they are me.

You are not alone on this path towards wellbeing. Many others walk in front, behind, and alongside you. They grapple with choosing the salad over the sandwich. They dedicate time for exercise. They struggle with their body image.

Body image is a phenomenon that lives in us all. We're each individually working towards a journey of wellness. And we're learning to fall in love with ourselves. Show some love for those who might not be where you are in this adventure of wellbeing. For the ones who started yesterday, for the ones who've been working for months but haven't seen results, and for the ones who haven't even started yet.

Send blessings to those who struggle with their body image, because we *all* struggle sometimes. Let's stop the self-sabotage and create a movement of self-love. Adore yourself.

Send positivity. Send good energy to your friends and family, to strangers, and to the world.

July 16th

I eat fresh made food.

Begin eating for freshness. Make fresh a goal. That's a great word, isn't it? **Fresh**. How does it make you feel saying it? What thoughts come to your mind? Plump, colorful fruit? Perhaps a clean kitchen that smells of bleach or newly watched sheets or a new sunrise.

When you eat fresh made food, you conjure the fresh feeling in yourself. You promote wellness in your body and in your spirit. It's so much lighter in your body when you consistently enjoy fresh made foods.

Make it a point more and more each day to avoid processed frozen dinners or fast food that uses ingredients that have been engineered. Fresh is best. Fresh, fresh, *fresh*.

I eat fresh made foods today.

July 17th

I win every day.

___

You are a winner. Every day you accomplish something, sometimes big and sometimes small. The trick to achieving your goals over and over again is to recognize your wins. Celebrate them, no matter how small. That joy from celebration and recognition will grow and grow until it becomes your normal feeling. And it should be. You are a winner. Someone doesn't have to lose for you to win. Happiness is your birthright.

Remember when you were growing up how great you felt when you learned to tie your shoe or ride a bike? Can you remember when you took your first steps? Maybe not, but you can imagine how amazing that felt. How grown were you the first time you stayed home alone or drove a car?

Glance around today and witness your wins. I win at creating my living space. I win at the productive conversations I have today. I win by eating well. I win by walking. By deciding to better yourself, you have accomplished greatness. You win, every day, always. You're a winner, baby!

July 18th

I eat at the best time of day for my health.

Time is of the essence. When do you find yourself in a delirious daze of hunger? After a skipped meal? Right before lunch? On the way home from work or school? When do you discover a surge of energy? Post-dinner? As you sip your morning green tea?

Today, eat at the best times of day for your health. Recognize your energy levels throughout the day and use your diet to supplement. Eat when you wake up and observe how productive your morning becomes. Grab lunch around noon to energize your afternoon. Slip in a healthy snack mid-afternoon to power you through rush hour. Sit down for a peaceful dinner at 7 p.m. Top it off with a sunset stroll to kick-start your metabolism.

Honor your body's natural rhythm. Align it with your diet. Like clockwork, it'll all start working in sync.

July 19th

I am worth the effort.

You're alive. Was that an accident? It wasn't. Everything happens for a reason. You are here for a reason. You're holding this book for a reason. You're fervently putting forth the effort to better yourself.

Before you question your work thus far by probing "will I ever reach my goals?" know that you are worth this effort. Happiness is worth the effort. When you exercise, your body releases endorphins - you're happy because you peeled yourself off the couch for a solid 20 minutes. And you need a clean diet to pump through that workout.

Better yourself because you love yourself. No one is like you and the world is better because you are here. You want to see yourself succeed. Put in the effort. It takes just as much energy to not do something than it is to do. Your physical, mental, and spiritual wellbeing is worth the effort. Put the time in and watch before your eyes your transformation towards a better you. No harm in trying, right?

July 20th

I bring loving attention to my arteries today.

Arteries carry blood to all parts of the body, delivering nutrients and sending oxygen to every cell. It is a closed loop system. Amazing, actually.

The heart pumps the blood. It is central to keeping you alive. When we eat foods that are fattening or have high cholesterol, we compromise our heart by clogging our arteries and disrupting the flow of blood… a flow that gives us life.

Our heart is also our emotional center. It is the part of us that loves and holds and measures morals and truest feelings. If the heart is our emotional center, then the arteries are our pen pals, sending love letters throughout our bodies.

When you bring your loving attention to your heart and arteries, you raise both your physical and emotional wellbeing. Eat right and think right, and think love.

July 21st

I am healing my body by eating well.

Feeding your system with a balanced diet of vegetables, fruits, and lean proteins, builds strength for your body and mind. Strength against stress, illness, or disease. The way to purify your body is by removing those impurities and replacing them with vitamins, minerals, and antioxidants.

Has anyone contracted bronchitis from broccoli? Nope, definitely not. Has anyone developed diabetes from daily donuts? Those odds are a little higher. In the United States, more people die from eating too much food than of too little. Yes, hunger is a problem, but over-eating is an even bigger one (and there aren't nearly as many charity events dedicated to it).

You don't need a butler with a silver spoon to eat good food. You don't need to live like a celebrity to shop in the organic section of the store. You simply should pick the bundle of broccoli over the bag of donuts.

It starts with one choice. Make the choice that betters your body, your spirit, and your mind.

July 22nd

I am in charge of my beliefs and choices.

Only you have the power over your life. You have the power to influence what you believe in and the power in each choice you make.

Friends, family, co-workers, and your community are beneficial resources. They provide advice, inspiration, and guidance in whatever situation. Everyone has an opinion, and sometimes that's valuable. Other useful voices help to center or pinpoint certain choices. But they do not control you.

Only you hold the ultimate influence in your beliefs and your life. No one can tell you how to live or think because nobody else is you. They don't see like you see, or think how you think, or speak how you speak. They don't have the same passions or interests. They don't have the uniqueness that makes you so incredible.

Today, know you are in charge of your life, through every belief, choice, and action. Rein in that strength. You are the leader of your destiny.

July 23rd

I eat foods from local cooks and chefs.

L ocal cooks and chefs provide the types of food that fit culturally for the region and using the best local ingredients. Local is a sense of your own intimate community. Your town's economy, school systems, roads, and services are all determined locally.

We watch & learn from the national and global areas because we all impact each other. However, the strongest, most immediate impacts occur right where you stand and expand throughout homes, neighborhoods, cities, towns, states, or countries. Basically, your wellness starts at home within you; then expands to your community.

Support your local cooks and chefs because ultimately, they support you. They are your best resource to connect quickly with the foods in your town that serve you best. Eat local.

July 24th

I eat at restaurants that promote healthful eating.

There are new health-focused restaurants and concepts popping up everywhere. Go there. Take the long way if you must. Vegan and vegetarianism are in; it's now trendy to be healthy. Lucky you-you're in style. This is a success for everyone because plant-based diets promote health and wellbeing (I challenge you to find any evidence to the contrary). Patronize these restaurants with your time and dollars. They believe in wellness like you do. Support your wellbeing. Make it a habit.

Treat yourself to the creative menu, often pieced together with local and sustainable foods. Find local cooks and chefs that want to support the community with homemade and handmade foods. Abstain from chains while establishing a healthy eating environment for you and your neighbors. Travel the extra miles. Feed your body and you'll feed your spirit. Eating well isn't always convenient, but it's almost always worth the effort.

"Anything worth having is worth fighting for." -Susan Elizabeth Phillips

July 25th

I practice friendliness.

Notice the kindness of others and then compare them to your behavior. Who is the friendliest, most amicable person you know? Why would you call them friendly? Are they helpful to others? Do the smile often? Are they a good listener?

Pick the qualities you admire and practice those traits. Be friendly to that stranger at the grocery store or the peer who annoys you for some reason you can't quite put your finger on. Give a compliment to the person you think doesn't particularly care for you. It's possible that you are not everyone's cup of tea, but be the honey to sweeten each sip.

By opening to positive feelings and uplifting others with kindness, you improve your own energy at the same time. Your mood elevates and up goes your body chemistry. Practice friendliness. Your connections to the world directly correlate to your wellbeing.

I enjoy lunch because I take a real "me" break from everything else to be present with nourishing myself.

I look forward to my lunch break. The time of day to break from your hectic schedule, back to back meetings, and swiftly approaching due dates. The time to sit down and nourish your body. Feeding your stomach the energy you need, to power through the rest of your day, and to take on whatever challenges might arise, massive or minuscule.

This lunch break is the most refreshing part of my day. It's a time of awareness. You can honestly consider your journey thus far and map out whatever detours arise. You can take time for yourself and that is time well spent.

Lunch is the meal that breaks up your day by allowing you to replenish your energy and refresh your mind. That precious half hour or so grants you the clarity of mind to pause and better pursue your journey of wellness. It's the wind in your sails, pushing you from a creek to a river, to an ocean of possibilities.

Enjoy your lunch today. Savor each bite. Swallow with care. Don't rush through this time; cherish this time. It's all yours.

July 27th

I eat my last meal at least two hours before I sleep.

Let's say you ate a late lunch or you came home from work late and missed your regular time for dinner. If you're planning to hit the hay in a couple hours, my advice to you is to forgo the big, unnecessary feast. We've conditioned ourselves to think we must eat three meals (or more) per day, placing a premium on dinnertime as our last chance of the day to slip in a balanced meal.

Food gives us the energy to function. If you're winding down the night, you don't need much energy to sleep. Save your late-night pizza order and tuck yourself into bed or munch on a light snack to send you into slumber. Wake up a little earlier and sit down for breakfast instead of grabbing a bagel for the road. I don't recommend a stack of flapjacks to make up for last night, but I see plenty of positives in a protein-packed egg and turkey bacon breakfast to jump-start your morning.

Skip the calories that sit dormant while you're sleeping. Don't starve yourself, but don't engorge yourself either. Retrain your mind by listening to your stomach.

July 28th

I am supported by my friends and neighbors.

As I've grown older, I've solidified my support system. During your high school and college years, you desperately search for friends, but as you mature, you see who truly has your back. Support from friends is magical. You can do no wrong in their eyes and they will love you through anything. It's rare to find that kind of love from one person let alone a handful. It's a love that transcends time. If you only have one friend who has your back, you have enough. To be encouraged by someone who wants to see the best for you and genuinely succeed – that's like stopping for gas on this road trip of supreme positivity. Take a rest stop and refuel your energy and positivity.

Today, thank your friends and neighbors for their support. Send them flowers or a gift card to their favorite store. Shoot them a text expressing your gratitude. Know that with your misfit group of partners-in-crime, anything is possible. Reach out to them and provide support when they need it most. Give and take is the recipe. Throw in a dash of love and a sprinkle of laughter, and you've got yourself a pretty sweet life.

July 29th

I wait 5 minutes before I satisfy a crunchy craving.

Crunch is oddly satisfying. The word itself evokes the essence of biting down for that glorious crack and resistance for a tasty release. Different from chewy, isn't it? Sometimes the crunch is thundering, like that bite into a thick, folded potato chip. Sometimes it's softer like popcorn, celery, or an apple.

Cravings are our body's way of wanting satisfaction. Check in with your body. You are likely not actually hungry when you have a craving, you just have a taste for something.

When you crave anything, wait it out. Use your mind to reason and see what's happening emotionally. Crunchy snacks are especially addictive. They're textural and animating. If you must, opt for the softer crunch for your wellness

July 30th

I am kind to the earth for providing sustenance.

Mother Earth – there isn't anyone who doesn't learn to respect their mother. She is the life-giver, the caretaker, and the future.

When you take from the earth and fail to give back, you break the relationship. The amount of waste that covers our land and fills our oceans will shorten the lifespan of this planet, and by association, all creatures. It starts with every individual. It starts with *you*.

Filter tap water instead of bottled water. Take magazines, newspaper, and plastics to recycling locations. Ride your bike to work or alternate transportation to cut back on fuel emissions. Upcycling is on trend; old barn wood is transformed into dining tables and antique cars are used to harness parts. When purchasing anything, delve into the history (and hope there is some).

With every peach, plum, and nectarine, we possess the power to replant. Kindness starts with thinking, realizing what's in front of you – and it's potential. Even that little peach seed can bring forth a fruitful harvest.

July 31st

I am rejuvenated.

You are living your own renaissance. With each step up a stair, a bite of an apple, and positive thought about yourself, you are birthing a new, healthier you.

Positive thinking leads to positive actions. Through those positive actions, you restore the health of your body, mind, and spirit. It's almost like uncovering the inner self that has always lived inside. It's an awakening of wellbeing.

A balanced diet of proteins, vegetables, and fruits can restore your energy. There's a childlike curiosity that unfolds – excited, inquisitive, and active. You restore that hunger for life. It's perplexing how the healthier you eat, the more you increase an appetite for adventure. You have a newfound energy to explore, learn, and do. Truly, it's confidence. Confidence to buy the plane ticket overseas, to throw a party in the middle of the week, to be your honest self.

Today, you are rejuvenated. You are alive - act like it.

August 1st

I am powerful. I matter. I make a difference.

Yes, this could technically qualify as three separate affirmations, but I'm a rebel. This is major reinforcement that this world would not be the same without you. Your presence impacts outcomes in an infinite number of ways. Your style influences and your behavior resonates.

Decide how to use your unique power right after you wake up; your power opens like a budding flower, greeting the sunshine, saying hello. When you take a call, answer a question, wear a smile, give directions, pay your bills, water your succulents, or walk the dog, your power is put into play.

All of our actions hold an interaction that affects the Universe. The Butterfly Effect is the concept that small changes can have large effects, i.e. a butterfly flapping its wings impacts weather conditions weeks later. Eat mindfully today. Everything you do matters to people beyond yourself. Say it, shout it, know it: I am powerful. I matter. I make a difference.

August 2nd

I am aware that healthful eating leads to a healthy life and vitality.

Eating well brings wellness to your body, mind, and spirit. You know this subconsciously as a fact, but maybe you don't always apply it to your life. Today you will bring this fact to the forefront of your mind. Stare it in the eye. Think about it over and over. Toss it over in your mind until you can say it backward. Eating good nutritious foods will make you feel good and bring you happiness. Carry out an effort to really know this.

It's not for other people's health plans. And it's not for tomorrow's diet. Healthy foods and habits give you energy. Improves your health. Clears your mind. Provides vitality. Be aware. First, you think it, and then you can act on it.

Today and every day from now on, keep this understanding with you always, like a mini shoulder angel whispering guidance in your ear. Listen and act accordingly by the choices you make. One meal at a time. One bite at a time. Starting right now.

What do you know now?

August 3rd

I am transforming my life.

Somewhere along my health journey, I stumbled upon courage and inspiration to transform my life into what I want it to be. Those two momentous ingredients come to you when your journey needs them most after certain lessons are learned. My biggest lesson hit me when I realized I was stressed because I believed through my education and social circles, that stress was the price of happiness. Happiness is the house, the car, the trips, the title. Overweight, nervous, with stomach and leg pains, I would cry easily at home and put on a suit of armor for my daily battles at work. Then, I had an epiphany – stressed out is *not* happiness. I asked my higher power for peace of mind. And I received it.

Transform your life into what you want. It may require giving up something superficial, but you can own the health and peace you desire. Transform your life. Start today.

"Ask and it will be given to you, seek and you will find, knock and the door will be opened to you."
- Matthew 7:7

August 4th

I am lighthearted and full of gratitude.

Weight is heavy. It can be burdensome, but it doesn't have to be. When you lift 100 pounds, it's challenging and if you use bad form, you will hurt your body. But when you use a pulley system, place it in a wagon, or even carry it in a backpack, the level of the burden changes significantly. And if you carry it in your car? Easy.

Consider your emotional burdens and physical weight the same way. Change your mode of transportation, or how you view things. A different perspective, which includes a positive disposition, will lighten your burdens.

When you're feeling low or disappointed at the weight on the scale or the reflection in the mirror, try saying:

"I am turning this heaviness into lightheartedness."

"I am grateful for this reminder for my health and grateful that I can start again."

"I am grateful for my progress in life thus far."

"I advance in the right direction overall."

"I am lighthearted and full of gratitude."

August 5th

I improve my life by making conscious choices to eat well.

Wave your goodbyes to the crash diets and juice cleanses because you want to lose weight. Change your intention and your method. Your healthy, happy weight will appear. Focus on your happiness and how your food can work with you to achieve that goal. Most people think of food as an afterthought; after they are hungry or after they've eaten.

Be strategic about your eating choices. Food and its reaction on your body is a powerful tool to achieving anything you want. Do you want a new job that requires energy and focus? Eat for it. You want to walk a 5K, run a marathon, or just walk up a flight of stairs without getting winded? Eat for it. Do you want a new house or car? Eat for it.

You need the energy to find the perfect house or car. Mental clarity to make the right decisions for your growth. Stamina to find and keep the job that will afford you the finances to fund your dreams. Use eating well as a major tool in your arsenal to improve your life. It is a secret weapon and a competitive advantage.

August 6th

I am strong.

Strength transcends your average weight room. Strength is both body and mind. Those two are inseparable; when you eat a balanced diet, and partake in daily movement, you establish overall wellbeing. Exercise is a stress-reliever and healthy eating can steer clear of depression and anxiety. If there wasn't already a reason to develop your body and mind along this journey of health, well, here it is.

You are already strong because you are reading this book. You are strong because you have chosen to better yourself. You are opening your heart and soul to new possibilities. I define strength as knowing yourself well enough to choose your emotions. I define strength as independence and creating your own path. I define strength as loving yourself.

Recognize your strength today. Really, all you have to do is look in the mirror; how easy is that?

August 7th

Today I bless my thighs and quadriceps, which power my stability.

Thank you thighs and quadriceps, knees and feet. Your legs do so much for you. Don't take them for granted. They need movement. Exercise keeps them oiled and fluid, ready for fight or flight.

Appreciate what they do for you. Your thighs and quadriceps have powerful muscles. Those hinges we call knees are their own study in physics and mechanics with pulleys as ligaments and an amazing technology of joints. And don't forget your ankles and feet. Would you have thought of toes? Try standing without them. They're a big help. Only the universe could be so thoughtful.

Start blessing your body and all its parts for how they support you. When you give love, you get love. Even and especially with your own body. Thank you, legs.

August 8th

I am faithful.

Being faithful doesn't necessarily mean attending weekly prayer. Sometimes being faithful means having faith in yourself. Today, find your faith. Having faith means thinking positively, and positive thoughts lead to positive outcomes.

Know that with each passage you read in this book, and with each turning of the page, you understand more about your health. Have hope that with each healthy decision you make on this journey towards wellness you grow stronger, smarter, and happier. If you do believe in a higher power, have faith that they are always listening. Have faith that the universe knows each thought, action, and movement you do and it reacts in return. Have faith in yourself that you will accomplish your goals towards mental, physical, and spiritual wellbeing. Have faith that it's all going to work out – because eventually, it does.

Have faith.

"…I have learned the secret of being content in any and every situation, whether well fed or hungry, whether living in plenty or want." – Philippians 4:12

August 9th

I focus on eating by avoiding the distraction of watching TV.

After a long day, all we want is to lie on the couch and zone out. This isn't something unique to this generation; it's a nightly ritual since televisions became a staple of living rooms. There are even "TV Trays" for you to sit down and enjoy your meals from the comfort of your sofa. This mix of dining and entertainment promotes mindless eating.

Resolve to separate the acts of eating and watching TV. Savor your meals, chew your food with thought, and swallow your bites before taking another. Find what you enjoy about your meals. Is it the citrusy lemon that accentuates your scallops? Do you love the heartiness of your brown rice? Understanding what you like about your meals and taking the time to truly appreciate them will allow you to pinpoint parts of your diet to accentuate, ultimately advancing you to reach your health goals.

By taking the time to eat, you'll not only enjoy your meal, but you'll be able to slow down with small bites instead of the mindless face stuffing. Increase your awareness by focusing on your food.

August 10th

I am thankful for my safety.

I'm safe wherever I go. Whether it's walking to my car at night or entering a party with people I don't know, I know that the universe has my back. Sure, it doesn't hurt to carry some mace in your bag, but I'm confident in my safety.

I am strong and brave. I can face any adversity. No matter what, I know I will be okay. I know that my neighbors, family, and friends will always protect me — emotionally, physically, and mentally. Not only do they protect me from harm's way, they lift me up and make me stronger. I'm safe with them because they create an environment for me to flourish. I'm thankful to live in a tight-knit neighborhood, where I know my barista's name and ask the grocery store clerk how her day was. I'm thankful to live in a neighborhood where I know it's a community of safety. It's a culture that breeds a safe space for freedom of expression. Whatever happens, I know my community will protect me and look out for me.

It's human nature to trust, so trust your neighbor and your coworkers. Trust yourself. You are safe because you tap into your higher power, and that will always protect you.

August 11th

I separate the events of eating and driving.

If you're driving, then drive. Today, if you look out your driver's seat, you have the high chance of observing a handful of other drivers behind a wheel, scrolling on their phones. Doesn't make you feel safe, huh?

I think we take the power of the wheel for granted. We turn up the radio, roll the windows down, and unfortunately occasionally check our phones at red lights. Cut out the distractions and focus on the task at hand. If you're late to work, you're late. Don't speed with the toast in your hand, jelly dripping down the steering wheel. Because when you turn around for that split second to grab a napkin, an airbag could smack you in your face.

Separate the events of eating and driving. Separate the events of driving and anything. It can wait. It always can.

August 12th

I recognize that eating out has significantly higher calories than home cooked meals.

Dining out brings forth the luxury of untying the apron. It's a time of relaxation. You sit back and sip your iced tea as you engage in conversation with your dinner dates, waiting patiently for your specially made meal. More often than not, however, the kitchen staff or chef work behind closed doors. Sometimes a window grants the view of the behind-the-scenes of your entrée, but you can never truly know the recipe. That is unless you make the recipe yourself.

When you cook at home, you control the oil, butter, salt, and sugar in your meals. When you dine out, you don't see the ingredients used in the process. When you cook at home, your food might taste differently because you're using fewer additives or processed ingredients. But, you're eating healthier.

Try and recreate a favorite restaurant meal on your own using organic or locally sourced ingredients. Add only a dash of oil and salt. Today, recognize that dining out has higher calories than dining in. Choose better. Choose healthier.

August 13th

Self-awareness frees me to see the truth.

There is no greater perspective than self-awareness. As we discover our emotions and our habits, we unearth a knowledge of self. We identify the person we want to be in the future, by knowing the person we are now.

Self-awareness takes a step back from your ego to clearly see who you are. When you honestly see yourself, you might notice you are quick-tempered, judgmental, or lazy. But you also might find you are empathic, genuine, or work best under pressure. With each shadow quality, there is a positive twist not far behind.

Self-awareness isn't a one-and-done step. It's steadily digging deeper, sifting through layer after layer, finding the new in yourself each day. You might never reach the axis necessarily, but you work your way slowly but surely to discover your wants, needs, and values. Learn something new about yourself today through self-awareness. Use it to enhance your emotions, interactions, and daily routine.

Once you freely see yourself through self-awareness, you see each moment with clarity.

August 14th

I choose harmony.

There's a harmony in the universe. You might hear it from the melody of sings the bird's chirp as you wake up. You might hear it from the pleasant conversation between strangers.

Harmony is around you. The balance of life has lived inside of you since you were brought into this earth. All you must do now is choose harmony.

Today, choose harmony in your wellbeing. You are harmonious because you support your choices and your actions. You create an environment of positivity in yourself. Find harmony through each thought, each word spoken, each bite eaten, and each action taken. Find harmony between all the processes that make you who you are as an individual. They each add to your personality and character, each action helping you to become a healthier person. You are balanced through harmony.

There's a song inside your soul, and it's harmonious. Turn up the volume, won't you?

August 15th

Today I focus on nutrition.

When we hope to become healthier, a large part of our goals are accredited to weight loss. We think healthier means skinnier which means happier.

Rather than focus on weight loss or the number the scale spits out at you each morning, focus on nutrition.

Focusing on nutrition means focusing less on weight loss. It's eating a balanced diet for you and your lifestyle. It's feeding your body with nutritious options to nurture your physical and mental health. Eating clean means clearing out waste from your body, but it's also a detox of the mind. You stop counting calories and start counting vegetables. You work more lean proteins into your diet rather than nix fried chicken or red meat completely. You find what makes you feel fantastic.

Focusing on nutrition is the most fundamental step in mindful eating. Of course, your guilty pleasures will patiently wait for you, but shift your focus to the foods that give you energy, a clear mind, and a happy body.

I am intentional about what I want.

The path of success must first start with an intention. Every successful person will tell you that to win you must first have a desire, intention, vision, hope, or dream.

Literature around this concept appears in numerous novels, such as Gary Zukov's bestseller, *The Seat of the Soul* or the late great Napoleon Hill's *Think and Grow Rich*. Mega-celebrity Oprah Winfrey lauds this theory, saying it changed the trajectory of her business – Oprah, a woman born into poverty who created an entirely new genre of television talk shows, as well as her own magazine and channel. So, this whole intention aspect might be worth a shot...I'm just saying.

It is a universal truth. Whatever it is you want to achieve, you must first clarify what you want. You have to really want it and think about it every day. Keep your intention firmly intact and the universe will undergo any and all planning that will bring your dreams to fruition.

A fleeting thought won't make a difference. A half-hearted whimsy will get you at best a glimpse of the infinite. A true dedication to your desire is what is required. Be intentional. State your goal every morning and every evening.

August 17th

I am bold.

How many times in your life have you worn muted colors, refused to say what was on your mind, or softened your personality for the benefit others? To deny yourself living out loud is to deny yourself the healthy mind and healthy body you so diligently seek.

Today, I challenge you to wear your most colorful adornment. I challenge you to say your true emotions when someone asks how you're doing. I challenge you to throw some color on your plate and dress up that kale salad with ripe red peppers, creamy avocado chunks, and freshly shredded carrots.

Once you decide to live boldly, you embrace confidence. You choose your own happiness over the happiness of others. You choose adventure over fear. Adopt a viewpoint where you prefer color. Life is too short to encompass a life of boredom.

"The whole life of man is but a point in time; let us enjoy it." – Plutarch

August 18th

I take 3 deep breaths when I have a sugar craving.

Take time and pause before you satisfy that sweet tooth. Cravings are a signal for something beyond the cupcake. Usually, the food is only a temporary stand-in for what really ails you. A sugary craving is the highest and loudest call.

When the craving hits you, take a minute to slow down. Take three deep breaths. Ask yourself, why do I want this cake? A chocolate bar or a taste for gummy worms? Your body doesn't need it and let's face it - candy is as far away from being made in nature as possible. Worms? Yes. Sour and sweet worms? Not in nature.

Take three deep breaths and figure out what's vying for your attention in your emotions. Feed that with your attention, not sugar.

August 19th

I recognize that my body is my container.

When we see our loved ones bash their appearance, we come to their defense by encouraging love – love that you see in them and that captivates their radiance each time they laugh, joke, or walk into a room. But how many times do we bash our bodies? Scorning the mirror, pinching our bellies, demeaning ourselves?

Take a few minutes out of your day, right now, to say something kind about your body. Your body is a container that holds your soul. Appreciate your body for being the vessel it is that sails your ship wherever the wind blows. Cheer yourself on through this wellness journey. Be grateful for your body. Uplift yourself. Love yourself.

With each vegetable and fruit, you fuel your body and flourish your health. Throw out a compliment towards your body when you wake up in the morning or when you exercise for an extra five minutes. Be kind to your body. You are on a magnificent path towards an existence overflowing with joy, and it's your form of transportation.

August 20th

I will monitor my salt intake today.

Salt is delicious. It is abundant in nature and a natural flavor enhancer. Salt makes everything taste vibrant. This is why it is overused in prepared foods. It acts as a preservative in some cases and makes food so flavorful that you are enticed to keep eating and coming back for more. Think about the tortilla chips at that Mexican restaurant. Hot, freshly fried, and coated in coarse salt, you finish basket after basket. The waiter tests you with each fresh basket, wafting the savory smell in your face as he sets it down in front of you.

I truly don't want to imagine a world where we take salt out of our food. Everyone knows those chips (and the margaritas) are the best part. However, the overuse of salt causes high blood pressure and leads to chronic diseases. Because it's hidden in a variety of foods, we often meet our salt intake for the day before we reach for the salt shaker.

Today, inspect some nutrition labels. Take part in some light reading. Taste your food for the saltiness on your tongue. Determine if you're getting the right amount and adjust accordingly. You make the ultimate decision about your sodium intake; it's not up to the waiter.

August 21st

I take time to enjoy the taste of each bite.

Watch how people around you eat. Seriously. Sneakily stare like a spy. Do they finish chewing and swallow before they take the next bite? Or do they chew a couple of times, swallow prematurely, and take the next fork full into their mouths? Before they even swallowed the last bite?

Now notice what you do. How do you eat? Mindful eating is the best path to long-term wellness. Because when you are mindful, you make positive conscious choices consistently.

Take time to enjoy the taste of each bite of your food. Slow down. Chew. Chew. *Chew*. Chew so you swallow with ease, many times. Gulp and pause for a few seconds to allow the food to travel. Make space in your stomach. In that time, taste. Savor the flavors that linger in your mouth. Create a new experience. Taste each bite.

August 22nd

I sleep well because I wind down for bedtime.

Sleep is extremely precious to our wellbeing. Please, please, *please* dedicate six to eight hours of your night to sleep. If you do not, ask yourself why not? Research sleeping habits and compare your own. It is important to recover your body and mind during sleep. Rest is mandatory. It is as essential as food and water; and like food, many take it for granted until they don't have any.

Treat your nighttime routine with more reverence if you have trouble sleeping. Develop a wind-down routine. Avoid the glaring screens of your devices or at least turn down the brightness. Swap the alcohol for tea. Take a warm shower or lavender scented bubble bath. Turn off the television and read. Not anything too scary or violent (might want to save the current events for mid-day).

Wash your face. Put some oils on your skin. Say a blessing for your family. Sleep tight. Don't let the bedbugs bite.

August 23rd

I renew myself every day.

Everyday is a fresh new beginning. Sometimes we wake up with yesterday's worries already weighing us down. We turn on the news, step on the scale, and review our texts and emails all within the first hour of the day. Of course, this gets us down and of course it's depressing. We're already overloaded with self-criticism, bleak world affairs, and a crowded schedule, all pushing us out the door and determining the day's communications before we leave the house. Lastly, we add caffeine to really amp it all up.

Do you see the insanity? Then stop, right now. Each day is new and fresh and made for your happiness and self-expression. Start each day with appreciation. Give your body a hug. Spend the first 30 minutes in blissful silence. Wait to check your phone. Renew yourself. Build up your arsenal of spiritual strength. Then, attack the world… with love.

August 24th

Today I give myself permission to be free.

I am unencumbered. I hold an infinite number of possibilities, simply waiting to be discovered. I have no limits. As a matter of fact, only the sky is the limit.

I can do and be whatever I want. I could declare today pajama day and wear my fuzzy slippers wherever I visit. Maybe I'll make it a movie marathon day, find a new documentary or tune in to a genre I've never watched. It's okay if I sleep in or spend the day catching up on old, unread magazines. I can purchase a new book, attend my place of worship, or sit on a bench at the park.

Be kind to yourself. Relieve yourself of your stressors. You deserve it. Give yourself permission to be free.

"When I discover who I am, then I'll be free." – Ralph Ellison

August 25th

My positive thoughts will create positive outcomes.

It's the law of attraction. This is a universal law, similar to the law of gravity. The law of attraction is that you attract to your life whatever you put your energy towards, either good or bad. It is not a one-time occurrence, rather a law always at work. Do you see people who always seem to have favor and everything works out? Or others who seem to be surrounded by misfortune? Life is unpredictable, but you're handed challenges because you're strong, brave, or witty.

The law works for everyone, at all times, always. Think about the gossips who are gossiped about or the bullies who end up in jail. But, it works both ways; there are servants who end up as Saints like Mother Theresa, the courageous who end up as heroes like Martin Luther King Jr., the peacemakers who go down in history like Mahatma Gandhi. These are all notable, but not unusual.

Your positive thoughts about your body and your dietary journey towards health can bring you positive outcomes, and it starts with a positive mindset.

"As a man thinketh in his heart, so is he." – James Allen

August 26th

I eat homemade food.

Who doesn't relish dining out? It's a treat when you sit down at a restaurant and are served on by caring staff. These restaurants usually produce the food in an efficient way to make a profit. This is especially true for fast food restaurants and chains, where they sacrifice quality for quantity. Mom & Pop places are often much more caring in the details of their preparation, taking pride in the customers' unique joy and satisfaction, not just for speed or convenience.

Speed usually comes at a cost of higher fat, salt, sugar, and processing. These items in large quantities work against your wellness. Store bought items have the same qualities as restaurants, with the focus on shelf life or mass commercialism.

Eat homemade and fresh made food as much as possible. Devote a weekend to making your own sausage, pasta, or salad. Go the extra mile and craft your own salad dressing. Look at you - you're unstoppable!

Eat homemade to promote healthier living and wellbeing. Do it for a week. Check in with your body on Day One and then on Day Seven. You will notice a difference.

August 27th

I understand that FEAR is False Evidence Appearing Real.

Fear is our biggest roadblock in life. It inhibits us from going forward, following our dreams, and too often keeps us from our life's purpose. The universe is created based on love. Over time we have conditioned ourselves that what we have is just too good to be true, so we let fear come into our lives.

Life is here for our exploration and enjoyment, but we've made it stressful. It's like your parents taking you to an amusement park with fantastic rides and fun games, but you won't play because you're afraid of the rollercoaster and the masses of people. You limit yourself, thinking it's other factors or people who are the problem.

What would you do if you knew the universe was actually *for* you? That ultimately you could not fail? You may have challenges and losses, but in the end, if you conquer your fear you will always win. If you don't quit, you win in the end.

Fear makes you think you're going to lose, be embarrassed, or fail at achieving a goal. It's false. You can do anything. There's ultimately only fear and love. Choose love.

August 28th

Today I will eat with my full attention on each meal.

Eating mindfully is a practice that develops over time. It provides you with growing benefits each day. The absolute value is improved physical and mental wellbeing. And it starts with one step. One bite. One day at a time.

Donate precious time today to focus on your meals. Start by thinking about what you will eat in the next 24 hours. Do you have the ingredients? Do you need to scour the World Wide Web or preview a restaurant's menu to prepare for future dinner plans? Focus on obtaining food and meals that nourish you. When you have it, give thanks for it. Admire the look, the smell, and enjoy the taste. Give all your attention to the meal in front of you.

Bite after bite, one at a time. Focus on your food for wellness.

August 29th

I am an influencer.

You are more influential than you know. We often look at our bosses, famous CEO's, entertainers, and any celebrity as an influencer. In reality, we are all influencers. No one is a deserted island; you are not unnoticed. Maybe you only have influence over a small circle directly. But because everyone you touch also touches someone else, your reach is much further than you realize.

You have power. Your life is a reflection of your choices. Others see you and are touched by your existence. You make a difference. You are an influencer.

"The most common way people give up their power is by thinking they don't have any." – Alice Walker

August 30th

I recognize the magnitude of conditions that must work in harmony to make each meal possible.

Take time to think about the symphony of nature that comes together to grow a plant, vegetable, or fruit. The sun, rain, and seasons have come together just so to produce a harvest. The harvest may be used to feed animals, furthering this chain reaction of nourishment for your consumption.

Stop taking this process for granted. Observe your next meal and contemplate the conditions, the farmers, the transportations, the shelving, and economy that came into the equation after Mother Earth.

This recognition will unearth a new respect for your food and its value to your wellbeing. Don't waste it. While it may seem like there are unlimited resources in your community, there are not. Millions around the world do not have the resources to feed themselves and ecosystems are changing. Your awareness makes a difference. You matter in the harmony of the system that feeds us all.

August 31st

I recognize my potential is unlimited; & so it is.

Imagine you are sitting along the shore of a river. There's a clearing in the brush and trees where you have a nice comfortable seat. You are reclining, sipping your favorite beverage, watching the flow of the river, as it travels downstream. Fairly peaceful with just enough activity that you know it's alive. An occasional fish pops out of the water, a bird swoops down for a visit. The sun is softly shining as the breeze glides off your skin.

Now as comfortable as you are in your world right now, that river is flowing with the unlimited potential of the universe. It's your potential to tap into and have anything your heart desires. You must leave that comfortable seat and put your toes in the water. Maybe wade into it until you are knee-deep. Feel and let the blessings that are yours grab onto you and touch your skin. When you really understand the bounty you'll fully immerse yourself. The river is unlimited. You can't even contain a fraction of what it has to give. But you can open yourself up wide and take the steps to move you to your blessings. Look inside your soul, and you shall find the universe.

My potential is unlimited; my cup runneth over.

Fall.

September 1st

I am right where I am supposed to be.

I went to the doctor yesterday for my annual physical. After all, it's around the time of back-to-school physicals, flu shots, and preventative vaccines. This is one habit I started many years ago when I was young, when most people I knew took their health for granted by only nearing a doctor for emergency visits. Splurge on the quality health insurance. Or, if you're lucky enough to be blessed with insurance from your job, take advantage of every penny of your coverage. It's a gift to your health to be preventative – not reactive.

The first thing they do at a physical is weigh you. My mood plummeted as my brain deciphered the number on the scale, slowly recognizing how much my weight had gone up. I went through the rest of the exam. Blood pressure? Normal. Heart rate? Check. Breast exam? Due for a mammogram, let's get that scheduled. What should I do about my weight gain? High, but within the healthy range. Simply watch your eating and move.

I decided to focus on the positives and take the weight gain as a call to action. Don't focus on the downs. You are right where you are supposed to be. Just keep moving forward.

September 2nd

I am constantly learning and evolving.

The curse of aging into adulthood is the societal expectation that you can't be a beginner again. Due to this, we skip out on new hobbies or activities we have yet to try for fear of embarrassment.

Being a beginner is vastly underrated. Oddly enough, there's a certain respect with the beginner title. When you're a beginner, essentially, you're a badass. You're fearless because you have nothing to fear. You roll with the punches and approach each day with wide eyes and a hopeful heart. Especially if you're in the company of fellow beginners, there is zero embarrassment, only excitement.

Learn something new each day. Challenge your brain and your body as you age. Break free from your know-it-all persona to stimulate your mind and spirit. You could be 100 years old and still not have read that lengthy novel or jumped off the high dive – so why not try the new, now?

September 3rd

I am aware that mimosas and Bloody Mary's are not actually breakfast foods.

This one goes out to my brunch buffs and Sunday morning stars. The license to drink in the morning, mostly from these morning libations, gave the world a whole new meaning for breakfast. They ease early flights and any holiday morning, including long Labor Day weekends and the like.

While these visually amusing drinks are lively and fun, they lower our decision-making for good healthy choices. You start your day off on a whim, and along with these drinks come hash browns, French toast, and every other decadent choice on the menu. You sip empty calories from the drink for a nice buzz, which leads to no discipline in ordering the meal. Then, the day is shot, so you start eating well tomorrow. Sound familiar?

Save these celebratory refreshments for special occasions, the ones where "cheers" is applicable. If you're doing it often, reassess its impact on your body. Eat a wholesome breakfast to start your day off on a positive note. Improve your wellbeing.

September 4th

I am prepared for tomorrow.

Remember when the new school year was about to start and you would shop around for stylish new outfits, a pair of shiny shoes, and fresh school supplies? I feel nostalgic watching the schoolchildren scurry around the colored pencils as they pick out bold notebooks. There was nothing like that Brady Bunch lunch box or Scooby Doo backpack.

Your parents prepared you for the upcoming school year. You had the tools and the uniform to tackle the classes. You packed your backpack with your pens and pencils. Laid out your clothes next to your bed. These were the good old days, weren't they?

Well, they're here again. Prepare for tomorrow, the week, and even the year ahead. Stock up on the groceries you need. Pack a healthy lunch. Keep a quick snack in your bag for emergencies. Look ahead and arrange your utensils in order. A builder doesn't show up on a site to build a home with an empty tool belt. Confidence in your actions stem from preparedness. Snag that cool new backpack and toss the pens whose ink runs dry. Prepare. Prepare. Prepare.

September 5th

I bring loving attention to my lungs today.

Take three deep breaths - your lungs just did that for you. They work 24 hours a day, 7 days a week, striving every day of your natural life. Giving you life. Driving your actions. Keeping you connected with your soul.

Your first breath is as miraculous as your last. Did you know that? God breathed life into you. You came screaming into this world, gasping for air. Each breath is the start of new life. When people meditate, they begin with deep breaths. When you need to calm yourself or relax, you go to your breath to inhale deeply and exhale softly. You breathe a sigh of relief. You breathe when you exercise, play an instrument, and give birth.

Your lungs grant you life. When you pay attention to your breath you find a stillness, and in that presence you are at your highest acuity state. It's there where you make your best decisions and are your best self. Honor your lungs for the oxygen to cleanse your brain, your bloodstream, and your heart. Keep your lungs clear so they will keep your mind clear and provide you the most pristine pathway to your soul.

September 6th

I am giving focus and attention today to my positive features and being thankful.

So often do we stand in front of our bathroom mirrors, picking out what we dislike about ourselves, leaving disappointed and upset. We then continue on with our days with a cloud over our head, reminding us of our insecurities and interfering with our moods.

Today, give focus and attention to your positive features only. Be thankful for what you do have, not scorn what you don't.

I like my big, brown eyes because they take in the wonders of the world. I see the sunshine around me, I wake up to the sight of my husband's face, and I am aware of my surroundings. I like my lips because they kiss my children goodbye and leave a stain on their cheeks. I like my strong arms and legs because I can move without gasping for air. What do you like about yourself? Be thankful for what you do have. No one else has your features. Own it.

September 7th

I create my own success every day.

Decide what you want to do today.

Do it.

Celebrate it.

Rinse and repeat.

You create your own success - others don't define your life, that's up to you. Keep your power and hold it close to you as you transgress along your wellness expedition. If you decide to walk to the corner today as your first step to exercise, do it. Don't compare yourself to someone who does three miles in 15 minutes. That's their journey. You succeed at walking to the corner - that's yours.

Draw in success by writing two things on your to-do list and work until you scratch them off. Don't drown yourself in despair because you had a list of two things and only did two. If it's the two you needed to do, then celebrate. Decide what you want to do next. Do it. Celebrate. Repeat.

You create your own success every day.

September 8th

I am thoughtful.

I have the best friends. Not many of them, but the few I have are incredibly thoughtful. They send me cards on birthdays and occasions and sometimes for no reason at all. They help me pack up and move without me even asking. They show up to all my events or occasions, no matter the distance. My friends always uplift me and encourage me. They are so thoughtful.

I, on the other hand, struggle to see myself as thoughtful when comparing myself to them. I could barely remember an event let alone a birthday, succumbing to the point where I've simply given up on trying. Originally, this stressed me out because I viewed myself as a bad friend when I forgot. Now I realize I don't need to feel bad because my heart and intentions are pure.

Being thoughtful isn't only greeting cards or meticulously wrapped gifts. It's loving, encouraging, showing loyalty, and being a good example. It's thinking about the world and your place in it. Think of love, peace, joy, happiness, and compassion. Then you, too, are thoughtful.

September 9th

I eat well to give thanks to the universe.

Eating well is developing a relationship with your food and your body. It's conscious. You connect with the origin of your food and the time spent growing, and how it traveled to your plate.

If you follow the idea that everything happens for a reason and that the universe has provided everything for you, then the universe has transformed the conditions to bring you your fresh made meal. Like stars aligning, the food you consume is a part of a bigger plan. Someone worked tirelessly to harvest your romaine. Another stood hours as a cashier to allow you to purchase your groceries. If you're dining out, chefs, servers, managers, and hostesses all came together to give you this meal.

Eat well to give thanks to this aligning of stars. The universe has conditioned each ingredient, each sprinkle of salt, and each second in time to bring you the meal in front of you today. Quite remarkable, huh? Thank your lucky stars.

September 10th

Today I celebrate my victories big and small.

I adore meeting new people. I look back on the times where I met a group of people who were career-oriented and civic-minded, both intelligent and spiritual. What a memorable combo. I celebrate that meeting still today. Why? We can't help but meet people every day, don't we? That's how we exist in this world. We may not exchange contact information, but we meet or come across new people everywhere - gas station, library, work, and even to the mailbox. What's not to celebrate?

I celebrate that I continuously meet a concentration of positive people. I celebrate that today, I am in a good mood because I remember those happy, inspiring people. I celebrate the friends who introduce me to positive voices. I celebrate the surroundings of those meetings. I smile when I reminisce on the good food we ate, the sunny day, and the cool temperatures. It was during the changing of the seasons. I even remember my hands clasped around my warm cup of tea.

Celebrate big and small things. It has a snowball effect to happiness

September 11th

I wait 5 minutes before I satisfy a craving for a nice glass of wine to give myself time to make the best choice for me.

Of all the occasions for a glass of wine, I find the most alluring are when I've either had a stressful day or an amazing one. Many of us have experienced that desire to run home and uncork a good cabernet, but after a few glasses, your night can transition from lighthearted fun to somewhat of a blur.

Cravings for anything are largely emotional. Take the emotion out of the craving. What really occurred? Today, wait five minutes before you satisfy your wine craving to grant yourself the time to make the best possible decision. Think about other possible outlets. If you're in celebration mode, call a loved one and fill them in on the excitement. Are you looking to relax? Breathe deeply in meditation or lose yourself in an entrancing hobby. Give yourself a few minutes to think about your choices. Be mindful about your body and mind; know how the two work together and choose positively.

What will you choose today?

September 12th

Today I bless my chest.

Show appreciation for each part of our body by giving it honor and gratitude. Your torso does a great amount of work. If you are an athlete or do resistance training, you know how important your chest muscles are and how it connects so much. Otherwise, you may take it for granted.

Honor your chest today for protecting your heart, for carrying your breasts, for displaying your jewelry, and for allowing you to function. You push out your chest when you're confident or want to show strength, so lift your chest high. Lead with your chest, it's more powerful than you think. Bless your muscles, skin, and flesh whenever you can. When you bless your body, your body blesses you.

September 13th

I organize my daily activity to ensure I have enough sleep.

Sleep is *sooooo* important. That's five O's. Rest is very, very, very, very critical to your overall health. That's "Very," four times. People brag about lack of sleep like it levels them with superheroes impervious to mere mortal needs. "I only get four hours of sleep" or "I haven't slept through the night in two years," or, I love this one, – "I get up to have a call with Tokyo at 3 AM every day."

Don't believe the hype. Your body needs rest and sleep just like it needs food and you need a paycheck. Sleep energizes your brain cells and improves your memory. Running out of fumes at work could be detrimental to your success.

You trudge into work and consequently feel horrendous, wondering why you're always sick. No, the barista didn't switch out that regular latte for decaf - you need rest. Plan your day accordingly. Shut off the television. Put your phone on airplane mode and get your seven superior hours. Wind down. Practice. Start tonight.

"I am sick and tired of being sick and tired." – Fannie Lou Hamer

September 14th

I take time to be still and feel the divine energy that is within me.

If you haven't tried meditation, try it now. Whether you're an expert yogi or a beginner sit down on the floor, cross your legs, and close your eyes. Breathe in through your nose and out through your mouth. Inhale and exhale on a count of three. When you breathe deeply, you can feel your body start to calm. You can feel the wind and the earth around you. You can feel the divine.

You originated from the universe. Space and time came together to map out your life. You are right where you are supposed to be; the universe planned it this way. This world, this city, this community would not be the same without you. You hold the same elements that make up our solar system. Recognize your divinity.

Today, take time to be still and truly feel the divine energy that is inside you. Harness that energy by acknowledging its presence. Once you do that, you develop a trusting relationship with the universe - and that's when the magic happens.

September 15th

I acknowledge there is a higher power offering me guidance.

Take time to recognize that there are endless forces at work in the world, most too impossible for you to understand. You are but a microorganism in a vast, vast existence. Do you understand fire? Gravity? Why people speak different languages or why the weather isn't the same everywhere? Why isn't the world flat? Why round and not square? How do acrobats and ninjas move their bodies with ease? Have you visited the Grand Canyon, Niagara Falls, The Pyramids or the Great Wall of China?

Call it natural laws, God, or whatever you want - but it's important to recognize that the universe is at work here. It impacts you so, that your mind couldn't even ever comprehend. It's limitless and wildly mysterious. Trust that the Universe knows. This place has been created for your happiness. Enjoy the ride. Follow the signs. Go with the flow. The Universe is guiding you.

September 16th

I will fully swallow what is in my mouth before I take another bite.

Remember when you were a child and you visited a petting zoo with your schoolmates? You fed the chickens, pet the goats, and giggled as the pigs joyously rolled in the mud. Those pigs also partook in some trough eating as well. They weren't eating; they were inhaling. Bites of food became breaths, each snort taking in the air as they filled their cheeks to the brim.

Sometimes I think we eat like these petting zoo piglets. Our stomachs become upset as we push food down without stopping for air or conversation. We refuse to lift our eyes from our plates until the contents have disappeared. And when do we suffocate ourselves with meals? When we're starving. Famished, we stuff our faces to console our stomachs.

Choose thoughtfully. Carry healthy snacks with you when you can. Throw a banana in your bag, eat a fiber-filled breakfast, and carry some nuts or granola to munch on throughout your errands. Stay on track all day. Chew each bite and swallow before diving in for another. Your stomach will thank you.

September 17th

Today I will ask for help.

You try to complete your tasks or responsibilities on your own so you appear confident to others, expressing your independence and flexing those "I got this" muscles. Becoming self-reliant is a benefit in some situations.

The reality is that nothing you ever do is based 100% on your own merit. Someone taught you your craft. Someone had influence in your life. Someone gave you an opportunity, a job, or career. Someone paid you, listened to you, and believed in you, even now.

Knowing this is liberating. We all need help at some point, if not all the time. Don't fear to ask for aid or some assistance. Help feels like support, love, and partnership. It is not pity or weakness. Asking for help also shows the other person how much you value them. Receive help today.

September 18th

I am building relationships with others who also want to eat healthy and to be happy.

Think about those people in your life that always want you to have another helping. "Is that all you're going to eat?" "You need some weight on those bones." "I only make this on special occasions!" Sometimes you feel compelled to eat more to make your grandmother happy. Or how about the friend who always gets dessert and wants you to pick one so they can taste both? And who doesn't love the life of the party who orders the next round for everyone?

While these people have kind intentions, you don't have to participate in anything that doesn't support your wellness. They want to make sure you've had enough to eat – ensure you have and thank them for their thoughtfulness. They want to enjoy your company longer so they offer another drink – order a sparkling water instead. Express your gratitude for their grace.

Recognize their kindness, express thankfulness, but keep your affirmations in the forefront of your mind. The more you're aware of your goals, the sooner you'll find your wellness. It's going to amaze you. Sit back and watch.

September 19th

I trust my intuition.

When your gut says "don't" in any capacity, trust it. The best move is your first thought. We doubt ourselves and in that doubt are decisions that are not your best. Trust that you made the right decision when you go with your intuition.

However, and I'll be frank, your desired results may not come from that immediate decision. Know that your intuition is giving you the best *overall* guidance. You need your trust and faith to persevere to the ultimate conclusion.

If you think you should turn right and you do, but the shortest distance was to turn left, that doesn't mean your decision was wrong. Maybe you avoided a car accident or traffic jam. Maybe you're about to meet the perfect contact or your one true love.

Trust your intuition every day. Especially when you are about to eat. What is your gut telling you today?

September 20th

I walk to destinations less than one mile away.

Do you ever run to the corner store to pick up something small, but you're not really running, you're driving? We're all guilty. It might only be a quick trip for items like aspirin or cotton swabs, but instead of burning emissions from your car, utilize the fuel in your body to power you down the street.

Combine those easy errands with your daily walking. You'll find an overwhelming sense of accomplishment. Sure, you only walked a couple blocks, but if you drove, you wouldn't have been able to stretch your legs or bask in the fresh air. You might even smell of nature when you waltz back into your living room, holding your aspirin and cotton swabs like an Olympic medal. Like that medal, your spirit is golden.

If you plan to travel less than a mile or two away, walk. Throw a backpack over your shoulder and free yourself from the restraints of the driver seat. Enjoy the time outside. Walk through the grass. Notice the flowers that grow in the cracks of the sidewalk. You'll earn your cardio and retrieve your aspirin. Be intentional and plan your walks.

September 21st

I take time to enjoy the texture of each bite.

There's a symphony of sounds around eating - the sizzle of garlic and shallots on a skillet, the spread of almond butter on hot toast, the crunch of a pita chip after it's scooped up hummus. It's like a living orchestra and you're the conductor. And with each sound comes a feeling. The flexibility of the celery stick, the hardness of an apple, and the softness of a raspberry.

Today, enjoy the texture of your food with each bite. Take in the sounds and smells, and round it out with that fifth sense of feeling. Is it soft and smooth? Does it sit on your tongue as you chew? Can your neighbors practically hear you chewing? Observe the texture in the tiny leaves of the asparagus. Notice the chewy texture of a rare steak. Make each forkful a mindful experience.

Immerse yourself in your meal. Relish in the experience around each bite.

September 22nd

Today I celebrate my friend's victories with them.

A support system of friends is like a quilt woven with memories and patches of time well spent. On the days you want to hide under the covers, your friends are there to wrap you in love and compassion. On the cold nights where you search for layers, friends are the ones who come in like a toasty fire and bring you warmth and comfort.

Today, direct some attention towards your friends today. Allow them to soak up the spotlight of happiness. Cheer them on for the milestones they've crossed. Express the love you hold for them. Show that you're their biggest and most loyal fan.

Friends provide us with encouragement, sympathy, and, if you're like me, a couple inappropriate jokes now and then. When you show support for your friends, they will show support for you. Give and take is what any relationship is about - give a little love when you can; take a little love when you need. Celebrate your friends today. After all, they have you as a friend, could they be any luckier?

September 23rd

I am free to express my authentic true self.

Be authentically you at all times. That word, authentic, has been thrown around quite carelessly. I adore that word and hope its meaning isn't watered down from over or misuse. Authentic means to have a verified origin. It also means to be true to oneself by honestly representing your true nature and beliefs.

I was raised in a culture where you kept your home life separate from your work life. You didn't want people to know who you really were, only to see the Employee of the Month in you. This is understandable given the years of oppression and bias that exist in the workplace even today.

But hiding my vivacious, funny, self wasn't me. I did not flourish. You cannot be truly happy when you are faking or restricting your true self. The true you, has admirable qualities and remarkable compassion, that needs to be shared with the world.

Free yourself to be you today. Be authentic.

September 24th

I spend more time on the outside grocery store aisles.

Here's one of the most health-altering pieces of advice: "all the food you need and for a healthy lifestyle is on the outside perimeter of the grocery store." Strikingly obvious, but I never noticed until it was pointed out to me.

The best way to shop is by priority and perimeter. Vegetables, fruits, and legumes first. Move on to meats and dairy. You'll have to pop in aisles for healthy oils and nut butters, or canned beans and rice, but stay focused.

There's no need to carelessly stroll down the aisles lined with sweet beverages or rows of chips. And the candy is too colorful not to call you if you visit that aisle. Stay on the perimeter and stay on track. That's where the good stuff is.

September 25th

I recognize the role that the earth plays in providing the food on my plate.

Everything you have has come from the earth at some point. The sun shined on the plants, which birthed your tomatoes and your heads of lettuce. The wind blows on the lilac as it grows and releases the scent as it sits in a vase in your living room, reminding you of peace each time a breeze passes. The rain waters the dirt and feeds the soil to sprout nourishment for all life. The bees buzz to each flower, pollinating and producing peaches, apples, and strawberries.

An entire ecosystem has created the contents of your life, especially within your refrigerator. Millions of organisms and circumstances on this earth have come together to produce the buffet on your kitchen table.

Today, recognize the role that Mother Nature plays in your life - beyond the "what should I wear?" conundrum. Nature is everything to this life. Throw some respect her way today.

September 26th

I understand that there is strength in being vulnerable.

We all need help. No one walks alone. You may see people you think have it all together. You know the type, the kind of people who seem like everything they do, every sentence or bat of an eyelash, bring some type of reward or recognition. We all have problems and challenges in our lives. It is meant to be that way. It is only within our struggles do we learn how to overcome; through experience, we develop strength. Like a broken arm recovering in a cast, every fracture rebuilds itself into a stronger bone.

When we fail to recognize the lessons in our challenges, we position ourselves for depression and self-pity, emphasizing worthlessness. This is wrong thinking. There is strength in being vulnerable when you search for the lesson and ask for help. It's the way of the world. What looks like strength isn't always strength – it's a cover-up, a façade, lipstick on a pig, a mask. Vulnerability takes courage. It builds stamina and a support system you would never achieve if everyone thinks you always have it together.

Find your strength. Be vulnerable.

September 27th

My food is medicine to my body.

Your body is sensitive. There are millions of cells at work that constantly give you life. They live under a microscope, out of sight and out of mind. Nonetheless, you are absorbing and reacting to elements around you all the time. When it's cold outside, you put on a jacket. When it's hot, you dab the sweat from your brow. When your nose is running, you wipe it. These are external.

Internally, there is an entire universe of activity that you respond to, however typically unconsciously. Today, start caring for your internal body as well as the external with what you eat. Food is medicine to your body. It's like the jacket or the tissue. It helps you to be comfortable and protects you from future harm.

Eat foods that make you feel better. It's the best medicine around.

September 28th

It is my intention to eat well.

We exist in a culture where everyone wants what they want, when they want it, and how they want it – did I mention they want it now? I originally would defend this nature, proving this endless want is a characteristic of normal human existence. But when you open your mind to a different perspective, you open the possibility of acquiring anything you want. We are spirits and souls living a human experience.

With this we can draw strength, patience, and guidance from our spirit and listen to our intuition and slow down. Have you ever seen a truly wise person whizzing around town? They take their time. Deliberate. Slow. Gandhi, Martin Luther King Jr., Mother Theresa, Dalai Lama, Pope Francis. Think of those who inspire you who you would confer with the title of truly wise. Embrace their ambitions. Mimic their attitudes. Create intentions that align with the ideals of the greatest minds in history.

When you set an intention to eat well, and slow down, then success follows loyally behind. Don't push yourself to limits you cannot reach; sit down and enjoy the ride. Be intentional and gift yourself the space of time.

September 29th

I use emotional triggers to my benefit.

Culturally we default to treating ourselves to something we consider sinful or decadent when we feel low or need a pick-me-up. Oddly, we use happy and celebratory reasons to indulge as well. The result? Over-indulgence.

With your new awareness toward achieving wellbeing, notice these times and employ your creativity to choose a healthier response to your emotional trigger. Don't end the bad day of work with a bottle of wine; sit outside with a glass of iced tea or hot cocoa. Or, use a joyous day of celebration to take a walk and relive the successes in daydreaming.

If you're indulging from triggers more than once per week, start to spread those out to monthly. Treats are good occasionally. Satisfy those triggers with life-affirming treats.

September 30th

I practice non-attachment.

When I first heard the phrase "non-attachment," I imagined a child running down the street, carefree and joyous. I wasn't too far off. Non-attachment is freedom. It's not holding on to circumstances, whether negative or positive. You become objective to all that surrounds you. It's knowing that everything will at some point pass, and you will keep living. You will endure difficult moments, but you'll also survive and move on to the happier times.

Life is constantly moving, you are constantly evolving, and you will always be a passenger along the ride. The obvious is that good and bad times will cross your path. While you can't always choose what will happen to you, you can choose whether to be affected by them. Once you envelop this feeling of freedom, you enjoy life a little more, with each giggle or tear shed. Think of non-attachment as not being stagnant. Time will keep ticking and you will keep moving. Challenge yourself and grow your mind. Find new opportunities as you work through the present. Know that it will always pass and you will always grow from whatever experience. Move forward. Be free.

October 1st

I activate the possible.

You create your life. You are just as special and likely as anyone else to do it. It's difficult to escape any rut when negativity seems to attract to you like a magnet - the job, a toxic relationship, money issues, or health issues. Life can be tough. I've been there. Interestingly enough, we *all* have. At one time or another, this short list above hits almost everyone. In this way, you are not special. You're no different than Steve Jobs or Mother Theresa. Everyone has adversity and you wouldn't want to trade their struggles for yours. Find your blessings in the battles.

The difference between people who find their way to happiness and those who don't is belief. You activate a better life for yourself by first believing that you can. From there, you act on it. One small step at a time. Practice continually taking these small steps. Celebrate the small wins. It's called progress. One day closer. One contact for advice. One healthy meal. One 30-minute walk. One job interview closer. One more day. Activate a turnaround and the upward trajectory to what's possible – your best life.

October 2nd

It is my intention to be a positive role model for others.

Role models are important influencers in our lives. Teachers, athletes, and parents typically top the list when someone asks you about your role models. But, we are all role models, no matter your title or station in life. We all teach value others can learn.

What you do matters. When you speak, someone is listening. The way you look attracts attention. The messages you send leave impressions, as surely as a drop of water in a pond leaves ripples.

Set your intention to be a positive role model for others. Because realize it or not, you are already a role model to someone.

"People will forget what you said, people will forget what you did, but people will never forget how you made them feel." – Maya Angelou

October 3rd

I eat healthfully for peak performance.

Your metabolism and ability to burn calories slow down over time. Knowing this, you can thoroughly adjust your eating and activity to balance the effect.

Eat protein to build muscle and carbs for your energy. Eat healthy fats and not saturated. Avoid processed foods; they slow the metabolism down even more.

As you age, eat less and cut down on portions. Yes, I said it; no one wants to face this fact. The math is simple and the body physics is obvious. You only need to eat for the energy to thrive throughout the day. Our culture promotes excessively eating more than what is required. To have optimal health, a weight that allows activity and vitality, and beauty inside and out, eat only what you need. Eat to satiety, not fullness. Eat nutritiously. Eat healthfully.

"One cannot think well, love well, sleep well, if one has not dined well." -Virginia Woolf

October 4th

My lifestyle promotes health and wellbeing.

Each time a relative comes to visit, I let them know my home is their home. My daughter stopped by one morning, while I was still in my pajamas and slippers. As she scoured the pantry, I informed her there were eggs and tomatoes and spinach in the fridge, or potatoes or even oatmeal. Her face scrunched up, perplexed. I was proud to say "you won't find anything unhealthy in this house."

I was impressed with myself in that moment because I realized I was transforming my positive choices into positive actions. I was walking my talk. She ended up discovering some saltine crackers from her last visit and made some peanut butter and jelly cracker sandwiches.

I learned that where there is a will, there's a way. When you want to live a healthful lifestyle, you will surround yourself with the environment that makes your success imminent. Yes, imminent. It's your life. Be well.

October 5th

I recognize society focuses on quick fixes.

It's easy to put a bandage on everything. We all desire the convenient speedy answer. Our culture is demanding, whether it's demanding time or convenience; we don't simply want it, we want it now.

Fast food replaces family dinner. Bottled water may be a time saver, but it is both economically and ecologically damaging. Texting versus talking overcomplicates our conversations to the point where the original message is lost. We accept pop culture articles and sitcoms over factual sources. Quick fixes work temporarily, but simultaneously create a future of problems.

Embrace your individuality and break from what the pack is doing. The input of time equals outcome of value. Ditch the quick fixes. Today, act slowly. Ease through the day. Take it one hour at a time. Dote on a recipe while making your meal. Think before you speak. Focus on the allure of slow actions. Recognize society focuses on quick fixes – and realize how you can be a leader for change in society.

October 6th

My spirit is contagious.

Ironically, one of the most memorable times I truly shared my spirit with others was the time I attended the funeral of a friend's son. I drove four hours on crowded highways to impart support and comfort in any way I could. What do you give to someone who has lost a child? There is no gift that is adequate. A donation? A plant? These are nice tokens of condolence, but each lacking in its approach. None big enough for the love I desired to show. She sipped her tea and revealed all she wanted in that moment was a pedicure.

Mani-Pedi's? Yeah, I can do that. We talked while our feet were scrubbed. We laughed while our nails were buffed. We commiserated in disbelief and took on some of her pain for her. In that moment, I saw how the spirit is contagious. When you approach something with love and thanksgiving it spreads to others. Its power is infinite and beyond meaningful, more than any other gift I could have given. In return, we were blessed by her faithfulness. I drove home in a daze, humbled by the event. I left with a new respect for life.

"My grace is sufficient for you, for my power is made perfect in weakness." --2 Corinthians 12:9

October 7th

I transmute fear into positivity.

We all are afraid at times. Whether you're slowly walking in a haunted house to prepare yourself for what's around the corner or if you move to a new city and don't know a single soul. Fear starves us from embracing our positive energy by feeding into our terror, keeping us from becoming strong, brave, and all around beautiful.

Today, convert your fear into positivity. Steer the energy you provide fear towards positive thinking. Illuminate your life with love, light, and happiness. If you should become afraid, remember the blessings in this life and remember your strength. There is nothing to be afraid of in this life that you can't handle. You are surrounded by love, from family and friends to your pets and co-workers. Love is all around. And fear is weak in the face of love.

Know that you are powerful. Know that fear is nothing compared to your transcendent power, your bright light, your happiness. To conquer fear is to fill a dark soul with sunshine. It's a solar eclipse of the soul – the moon can't stop the sun. Don't let fear stop you. Positivity is the way.

October 8th

I am resilient.

Be resilient. Resilience is a word that is personal and not yet overused enough to lose the beauty in its meaning. It means to bounce back in a soft but firm way that does not harm others, yet strengthens you. It's not the "dust yourself off and pick yourself up by the bootstraps" type of tough love.

Resilience is fearlessly trying again at life when it lets you down. It's more like those precious mornings when you played on your bed as a child, bouncing up and falling down; and with each push, you bounced back up and kept jumping. The best visual is like dough. When you press down on it or stick your finger in it, it rises back to original form. It won't be harmed but dented for a short time. Remember the Pillsbury® Doughboy? Someone would stick a finger in him and make a hole. He would giggle and return to normal. That's resilience.

October 9th

I acknowledge that unhealthy eating leads to low energy and chronic diseases.

The first steps to solving any challenge is to recognize it. People put on blinders and rose-colored glasses when they don't want to know the truth.

"Unhealthy eating leads to low energy, sickness, and disease." Believe this and know it in your bones. Throughout these changing seasons, it's time to focus on the vitamins, minerals, and nutrients you absorb from each meal, snack, and beverage that enters your mouth. Build up an iron wall of defense from antioxidants and Vitamin C to fight disease. In return, you'll acquire energy and health, becoming the envy of your sniffling, sneezing peers.

Unhealthy eating leads to low energy, sickness, and disease. Do your own research. Investigate like a disease detective. No matter the season, it's important that you eat consciously and make choices with your eyes wide open for the betterment of your health. Cultivate a healthy lifestyle with each bite. Give your utmost attention to your wellbeing and you can control your wellness destiny.

October 10th

I believe everyone should have access to fresh and homemade food.

When I watch my husband prepare a meal from scratch, I am astounded by the gentle care he uses to handle each ingredient. He takes his time, he dotes on the recipe and uses his passion to create something that will nourish us. Homemade food assists us in reaching ultimate wellness. Now, we have become engrossed with day to day activities and in our rushed stupors, we depend on large corporations to feed us and find we are at the mercy of these companies, taking in their preservatives & additives willingly. People seem to be less happy with their food selection and it shows through their feelings of sluggishness general unhappiness. Fresh food, on the other hand, improves our moods, our bodies, and our spirits.

Homemade food, or food made from scratch, has that *je ne sais quoi* not found in your cellophane packaged TV dinner. True homemade food is fresh ingredients, hand prepared. Get your hands dirty. Make a mess of the kitchen. Have a food fight with the leftovers. I feel everyone should have access to the advancements that homemade food provides.

More natural. Less chemical. Feel better. Look better.

October 11th

Today, I focus on drinking more water.

Water. It's essential to life. It's where you develop as an embryo to an infant, it's where you learn to hold your breath, it's where you play. There are few things as pure in life as a baby splashing in the water – their eyes large, mystified, and curious. This thing, this substance that's seemingly everywhere, is vital to our wellbeing and our health.

The brain and heart are about 70 percent water, the lungs around 80 percent, and the muscles and kidneys aren't too far behind. Our bodies are literally made up of water; no wonder why you're parched after that hike, run, or yoga class. *Hello!* You're sweating out the substance that makes up your entirety! Water flushes out toxins, boosts your immune system, and increases your energy. And the more you drink, the more you'll gain - smooth skin, silky hair, smaller waist.

Today, I will steer my focus towards drinking more water. Two liters. Eight glasses. I will keep an eco-friendly water bottle in my bag, by my bed, and on my desk. I will sip joyfully. I will replenish. I will live.

October 12th

I am aware that a whole foods diet improves my wellbeing.

Whole foods are those considered closest to nature. Food in their purest form. Fruit, vegetables, beans, and legumes. Whole foods are not processed into a similar substance, like applesauce. The whole food is the apple, core, seeds and all. The applesauce has potential to be whole, that is if it's not topped with processed ingredients that aren't whole, like sugars or additives.

Whole foods are the healthiest for your body. What comes from nature is specifically meant for anyone who wants to live a healthier and happier life. What comes from processing is meant for commercialism.

Stay aware. Be well.

"I am seeking. I am striving. I am in it with all my heart." – Vincent van Gogh

October 13th

I fill nighttime snacking with fresh vegetables and fruits.

We all have our nightly routines. Some of us meditate on our comforters. Some might take a hot bath surrounded by candles. Some of us (ahem, me) dance around the kitchen in search for a midnight snack.

If you're antsy and looking to munch on a snack during the small hours of the night, opt for fresh fruits or veggies. They're lighter than foods like toast or cookies. They boast antioxidants and vitamins, as well as a high water content. When I choose a bowl of berries over popcorn, I notice I wasn't truly hungry in the beginning. I simply wanted a snack to send me off to sleep. But when you finish the artificially flavored microwave popcorn, you might be too late to realize this.

Once the evening hits, if you're in the market for a snack, choose fresh produce. You'll be free of post-snack guilt, feel lighter, and hydrated when you wake up.

October 14th

It is my intention to let my inner strength be a beacon for others.

Believe it or not, but someone looks up to you. No, I'm not kidding you. Right now, they think to themselves, "what would _____ do?" People admire you, so set a positive example. Set an example of strength and inspire others to be strong.

Look how strong you are already, you have decided to better your health and wellbeing, and it takes strength to change. Whatever you do today, provide an idol for your fans. Use your voice when needed and the shy teen in the corner who sees you could be inspired to do the same. If you see someone being harassed or bullied, stop it in its tracks. Stand up for those who struggle to stand up for themselves so that one day when they think of you, they can.

Be a beacon of hope, a lighthouse that shines light out into the vast sea. Offer up a sense of direction. You are a symbol of bravery and positivity; recognize that, because everyone else does.

October 15th

I give thanks for the farmers who harvest the food.

Imagine yourself in the rolling wheat plains on an early morning. The rooster crows from the rooftop, signaling it's go-time. You rise before the sun to start your day. Feeding the animals, harvesting the grains, tending to the strawberries or tomatoes that have yet to bloom. You spend your whole life doing this not necessarily for the money, but for others. You do it, day in and day out, to simply see the joy on a someone's face as they sink their teeth into a crisp apple.

Give thanks for the farmers who harvest your food. It transcends the produce aisles; this is someone's life and they have the ultimate responsibility to feed you. Forget the mass corporations or fast-food joints. Honor those who plant the seeds, water the soil, and dust off the dirt. They hold an innate patience to see through the growth of each ingredient in your salad. And with our instantaneous world, patience is not common.

Show a little love to the women and men who are often unrecognized. They do more for you than you'll ever know.

I will replace ordering dessert with a nice warm cup of coffee or tea.

A friend of mine specially orders a specific cake each year for her birthday. The vanilla cake is thin, yet piled along endless rows of caramel, and finished with a cream cheese frosting. Each year, she plans for this heavenly cake, inviting everyone over for a slice. I believe this is the intention of dessert – to be saved for those extraordinary days and celebrations of life.

Desserts are tempting. They enchant us with edible flowers, gold trimming, or a shiny glaze. Since these foods are burdened with high amounts of sugar and fat, they gain a higher count of calories. With all the processing of foods now, dessert can quickly sneak up on us to work against our healthy lifestyle goals.

Reserve desserts for special occasions. Treat yourself to a soothing cup of herbal tea instead - Chamomile to soothe your nerves, Echinacea to treat that cold, or Rooibos for an antioxidant upgrade. All we really want after dinner is something to comfort us, something to round out our day. Encourage yourself to pick tea with honey over that scoop of ice cream. Set aside desserts for the moments of celebration and happiness. Bypass the sugar high for an elevated spirit.

October 17th

I practice patience.

"God, help me. Thank you, higher power, for each obstacle and opportunity for me to practice my patience." Each time I'm confronted with a fork in the road, I say that prayer aloud. Like when you read an email about yet another delay in a work project. You think to yourself, weren't we clear? Didn't we have minutes reflecting the urgency of the deadline? Didn't they understand the series of events following that are reliant on the first domino to drop?

What do you do when things aren't going the way you planned or want them to? Bumps in the road happen to everyone, regardless of how well planned or well timed. Maybe you left the house early for your appointment, but construction or bad weather still makes you late. Maybe you've saved your money, but unexpected repairs or injury set you back.

First, breathe. Three big belly breaths, with four counts in and out. Then, recite the prayer above in the first sentence. Finally, rest right there. Put it in God's hands. You've done your best; now give him the rest. Congrats on your first patience practice. Class dismissed.

October 18th

Relationships are important to eat healthy.

We are not meant to be alone. We express our humanity and our love for life through our relationships. Relationships are fundamental. It's why extended solitary confinement is one of the cruelest punishments imaginable. It's why Eve followed Adam and why it takes two to procreate.

There is an ancient saying, which claims you are who you are through your relation to others. Think about it. Who are you? Your answer typically starts with a definition of your relationship to the world. I'm a mother or father, a daughter or son, teacher, executive, chef, athlete. You exist beyond a title and in a universal understanding.

Surround yourself with people who support you, who want you to be your best. That is true love and compassion. If they want you to fail or like you unhealthy so they can feel better about themselves, then place that relationship in its correct position that aligns with your health priorities.

October 19th

I connect with my true self.

I heard in a sermon that when you pray, you're speaking to God, but when you meditate you open the space for God to talk to you. Sit with that for a minute.

Those of us who pray have been taught its importance along with praise and worship. Those in the West are only now learning the ancient wisdom and importance of meditation. It's where your truest self is revealed.

Don't talk at your higher power. Your higher power is *within* you. Speak with your power. Give & receive. Have a conversation. Reject the pleading or asking for what you want. Connect with your inner wisdom to learn how to achieve what you want. Go after your divine inheritance. It's waiting there for you to connect.

October 20th

I will have one meal serving for dinner this week.

Food is necessary, but we have transformed the consumption of food to a sport and a luxury. Hot dog eating contests and stuffing our faces until we have to unbutton our pants hamper our progress towards optimal health.

Some people eat to live and some people live to eat. Change your mindset to eat to live. Only eat one serving at mealtime. This doesn't mean load your plate sky-high and call that one serving. Create a meal with portion control in order to leave you satisfied in your stomach. Your mind might plead your taste buds to return for round two. Listen to your body. Are you really still hungry, physiologically?

Curb those cravings and stop at one serving. Give thanks for the ability to make good decisions. You can always grab a better choice in an hour or two for a snack if your hunger returns. Let your body tell your mind, "I'm satisfied already. I want to be healthy, so I stop at one serving today." Listen to your body. That vessel for your soul has some stellar points.

October 21st

I do small things every day to provide vitality for myself and for others.

Every minute has the possibilities of new beginnings and a fresh start. We wait until tomorrow, or the first of the month, or the dreaded Monday to start a new project. It's time to break the "tomorrow" habit. It's unnecessary. Procrastination. An excuse. You can take the opportunity within each second of the day to make a new decision, whether it's first thing in the morning or before tucking yourself into bed.

Choosing a healthier lifestyle for vitality, energy, and endurance begins with one step. Even if you do not start with a new habit in total, make one conscious choice that is healthy and positive. Maybe it's eating one piece of fruit. Maybe it's cleaning out your closet to donate clothes. Maybe it's something kind to the earth, like not letting the water run, drinking out of a cup that doesn't get disposed of in a landfill, or purchasing a household cleaner that is green, sustainable, or not tested on animals.

Small steps of thankfulness and awareness will make big differences in every corner of your life.

October 22nd

It is my intention to live fully.

What is living fully? I believe it's a balance of enjoyment and a healthy lifestyle that lead to longevity. It's about absorbing the best of everything. It's reducing the stress and angst while magnifying what brings you joy.

Interest yourself. Immerse your mind in art, in acts of kindness, in family and friends. Immerse your body in plates of healthy goodness. Immerse your palette in something new.

Leave your comfort zone to journey to the unknown. Learn as much as you can. Each day interprets an unfamiliar language, find out the name of your neighbor, or look on a map and find a country that once seemed foreign. Take an interest in the new to increase your self-awareness. And always share; share what you learn with others to find a sense of fulfillment.

Living fully is up to you. It's self-interpretation and application. Strive for happy.

October 23rd

I am my biggest supporter.

Be your biggest fan. Don't worry about sounding conceited, vain, or arrogant. Talk yourself up. Today, make complimentary statements about yourself to others. Go on. Practice it. "I love this outfit, don't you?" "I have such great energy." "I'm really good at..." (Here, insert math, art, leadership, or whatever).

Most of us fail to admit our greatness because we fear others will think we're full of ourselves. Too often, we intensively worry about what others think. Women are especially guilty of this, like over-apologizing or keeping quiet to look small to the world. The people who do toot their own horn are regarded as alpha men; running companies, rich, big houses, living their dream. Call them a toot, but they have what they want. *They* are their biggest fans.

Pat yourself on the back. Let others know your strengths. You don't need to be arrogant or braggadocios. Just be honest. You're a certified superstar.

October 24th

I eat healthier when I focus on the meal as I am eating.

How often do you multitask? While some portray multitasking as a virtue, recent studies have shown that the grass isn't necessarily greener on the multitasking lawn. It's best to be fully present for the task at hand, not half-heartedly working on your to-do list tasks simultaneously.

When you sit down for your next meal, actively decide to be focused on the meal. Do not multitask. When was the last meal you ate when you weren't watching TV, reading the paper, texting, or talking on the phone? We've taken the *meal* out of *mealtime*, focusing only on the *time* to do something else. Choose to honor those sacred minutes around your relationship with food. Your wellbeing and health is a priority now.

At mealtime, focus on the meal. Taste the varying flavors of your roasted vegetables and pan-seared salmon. Squeeze fresh lemon and watch as its acidic juices are absorbed. Close your eyes when you chew and focus all your attention on your meal. You'll instinctively eat better and find confidence in your breakfast, lunch, and dinner routines. When you choose to focus on your meals, you choose gratitude and bliss.

October 25th

I make thoughtful decisions.

Health is about taking little steps every day to better your wellness. It's the choice to move in a direction of wellbeing through thoughtful decisions. You notice what foods make you feel energized and improve with each positive choice. Small but mighty, these positive decisions make way to other positive decisions.

Imagine you purchase a head of romaine lettuce. With this romaine, you have made a small decision that could impact the rest of your week. It can become a salad, a layer on a burger or maybe you make lettuce boats to sufficiently scoop up your Tex-Mex instead of nachos. It all starts with one step, one decision, and one choice to determine a positive outcome.

Start by picking one positive action or influence. You will evolve into a being made of positive choices, each cell coming together, creating a healthier, happier you. It starts with one positive decision. What will your thoughtful decision be today?

October 26th

Today I focus on healthy fats.

Now I'm not a nutritionist, doctor, biologist, or anything in a lab coat, but I do know there are healthy fats and unhealthy fats. Today, focus on oils with healthy, unsaturated fats like vegetable or olive oil, from seeds & nuts, and even some fruits like avocado. If you're really feeling adventurous, test out the waters of polyunsaturated fats and omega-3's found in seafood like salmon or oysters.

The not-so-good fats to avoid, the ones to avoid as best as you can, are called saturated fats and trans fats. Saturated fats, which are solid at room temperature, are found in butter, shortening, and coconut oil. These partially hydrogenated oils are used in deep-fried fast food, donuts, margarine, and processed snack food. Say no to trans fats.

Healthy fats are your friends. They improve your heart health, provide immunity, promote daily activity, and strengthen those vital organs. It fights cholesterol like little cholesterol ninjas, slicing blood clots in half. The good fats keep you fuller, longer. Eat the good fat today and break the bad reputation.

October 27th

I turn off the TV while I eat.

In France, bistro tables line avenues for people watching and city viewing. In China, chopsticks increase the focus on your meal while you're eating, maneuvering each small bite into your mouth. In America, we plop our butts down on the couch with our TV trays to transform our dinners into entertainment.

I find a distinct relation between this televised dining and America's overall health. We boast the highest rates of diabetes and obesity, while we spend hours on our futons. Televisions increase mindless eating. You're distracted by the drama or comedy (or both) and before you make it to the second commercial break, you've finished your plate of food.

Find the sweet solace of the moment between you and your meal. It's a relationship, so treat it as so. Would you ignore the conversation with your date because you tuned in to your favorite show?

If you need entertainment, find it elsewhere. Open a window and look outside at the world around you. Spare your eyes the radiating blue light for natural sunlight or soft candlelight.

October 28th

I honor myself by wearing clothes that are comfortable and flattering to my body as it is today.

Without always realizing it, we punish ourselves when we are out of what we view the ideal state. Instead of wearing or buying the size that fits, we squeeze into an outfit so we can say we did. Rationalizing in our mind how it makes us feel better about ourselves.

You are not your dress size or pant size. You are so much more. You deserve to be comfortable throughout the day. You should feel good. Not stuffed and stifled into your nearing-vintage jeans because it's what you used to wear, but unleashing confidence in the blazer that makes you feel taller. Don't punish yourself by wearing an outfit that is too small. Accept yourself and love yourself for where you are today.

Be comfortable. Breathe. Move freely. Promote your own happiness. Don't imprison yourself in hate.

Love yourself. When you love yourself, then no matter the size, that love will shine through to others. You have to love yourself.

October 29th

I am aware of the importance of rest.

Everything ebbs and flows. Rest is important. It is as important as any activity you can do. You cannot be at peak performance without taking time to rest, sleep, and unwind. This rejuvenates you, keeps your mind sharp, and your words kind.

When you work out, you tear muscles and must allow them to rest and repair so you can come back stronger. When you are up working, cooking, and living for 16 hours a day, you need that eight hours of sleep to rebuild your body and mind.

Send a silent blessing to help those who brag about working 80 hour weeks and only needing 4 hours of sleep a night. Lack of sleep is not optimal to living a healthy life and being your best. Stress, ulcers, depression and so many more negative consequences result from a deficiency in rest. Be a leader in this area of your life. Bring awareness to rest.

October 30th

I recognize that I create my self-image and it is positive.

Remember when you were young and you curated this idea of your future self? You couldn't wait to grow up and be that person. Guess what – you're that person. You have the choice to allow your imaginations to become reality, so be that person.

Pull out the old drawing board and illustrate the self-image you've always wanted to see in yourself. You are the artist behind your life's masterpiece. You have matured and aged into a cultured, intelligent being. Everything you do oozes style and sophistication. You're cool, calm, and collected.

Find that childlike wonder and excitement for your life again. Harness the positive, hopeful image you've dreamed of over the years. You are the only one in control of how you view yourself – so make it a good one.

October 31st

I am aware of my fears.

What do you fear? You can't overcome your fears if you don't admit them. Are you afraid of being alone? Embarrassment? Failure? These are the top answers you hear. If everyone has the same fears, then why be afraid? These occurrences are normal and there is no shame in being alone, embarrassed, or failing.

You won't know how to have a healthy relationship until you can have a healthy relationship with yourself. The path to success is built on failure. And embarrassment is a synonym for failure. A misstep is just a trial run for success.

Be aware of your fears. When you illuminate your fears, they dissolve. You can't fight the darkness, but you can turn on the light. You don't win by fighting hate with hate. Only love wins. You can't fight loneliness with overeating. Your wellbeing wins. You can't fight failure with overmedicating. Only continued energetic pursuit of happiness wins. Be aware of what you fear. Then, turn on the light.

"For God gave us a spirit not of fear, but of power and love and self-control." – 2 Timothy 1:7

November 1st

I am beneath no one and superior to no one.

With cameras that are built in to face us as we pick up our phones, it's difficult to not grow a big ego. As we birth new generations into this selfie-era, we are confronted with the balancing act of confidence versus cockiness. Reality shows and social media give us a bird's eye view on how we think we *should* be.

The Internet and media have a strange cycle of self-perception; we compare ourselves to others, sometimes we think we're better and other times we think we're worse. Know that you are not superior to anyone, but you are also not beneath anyone either.

We are all humans on a journey. You are a human on a journey towards health and wellness of the mind, body, and spirit. You have plenty to learn, but you've also accomplished greatness. Find the balance in your ego and in your surroundings. Know that all human beings are equal. We all are born and we will meet the same inevitable outcome. You are unique and different. Harness your uniqueness and know you stand out in this world. That doesn't make you any better or any lesser, but it makes you incredible. Just the way you are.

November 2nd

My quality of life improves every day.

Quality of life. What is that? How do you assess the quality of one's life? You do not and cannot assess that; it is immeasurable. That's where we get caught up. The lives or habits of others are not yours to judge. The more you assess the lives of those around you, the more other people's opinions of you impact your happiness.

You can only assess, impact, change, grow or create your *own* quality of life. How do you measure it? On the surface, it may be how much money you make or the popularity points you gain by snagging the perfect mate. Only when you go deeper and understand your true self, do you assess the quality of your life. You assess it by the circumstances or ideas that are not fleeting. Like your purpose, compassion, or how much contentment & peace you have in your heart.

People and jobs come and go. Your soul is infinite. Realize more of the true you every day and the quality of your life will grow every day.

"If I cannot do great things, I can do small things in a great way." – Martin Luther King Jr.

November 3rd

I eat to satisfy my hunger.

Recognize this… Eating isn't an action to satisfy boredom, it's a need. If you are full after you have eaten a meal, you have overeaten. Your body works best when it has the right amount of the right food. You know when you are eating too much. In your mind, you say, "I shouldn't" or "I know I don't need this." Well, you're right. Since you are practicing more awareness, you, in turn, start the practice of following your best decisions.

When you overstuff a pillow, it's not comfortable to rest your head. If you fill a glass to the rim, it's difficult to maneuver those initial sips. If your luggage is too heavy, you'll hurt your back *and* pay extra fees at the airport. I could go on.

Think of your body the same way. Stuffed is not good. It weighs you down, literally. Eat to satisfaction. Then, stop. Practice control of your eating to control your health journey.

November 4th

Gratitude is the magical key to happiness.

What are you grateful for today? Sometimes when work, family, money, or body image issues dominate your focus, it's difficult to remember to be grateful. When you focus on the many pressures in your life at once, what you do have in your grasp suddenly blurs. But, if you pinpoint your focus on your true goals, the ones you scribble down on post-it notes and stick on walls around your house, you'll find gratitude will flood into your life, washing away the anxieties of yesterday, today, and tomorrow. Those moments of gratitude feel like happiness. They are happy.

It's really impossible to sit in gratitude and be unhappy at the same time. So, practice. Whenever you feel discouraged. If today something goes awry, just say the word "gratitude." And think of it. Your day just got better.

All together now: gratitude.

November 5th

I recognize that eating well is the best medicine for the body.

In today's society, we focus on cures for our pain and disease. We have vaccines that protect us from past epidemics, and we have created cures for many diseases.

There is no cure as certain as food. Food and your environment are the best medicines for your body. Prevention is key. There is no need for a cure if you are healthy. Change your mindset. Change your lifestyle to improve your health and wellbeing. If you're struck with a headache, eat foods that are soothing, cooling, and reduce stress. If you feel a cold coming on, stock up on sources of Vitamin C or Zinc.

Find the things that keep you healthy. Recognize and prescribe yourself the best medicine…. Proactively.

"The doctor of the future will give no medication, but will interest his patients in the care of the human frame, diet, and in the cause and prevention of disease."

– Thomas Edison

November 6th

I practice humility.

Every person has worth and value. People have more in common than their differences. Easily one would feel humbled in the presence of an iconic figure but those more pedestrian can also instill modesty.

It's easy to separate yourself from others based off of appearance, talent, or intelligence. It's easy to be impressed when you meet a brain surgeon or a celebrity. But what is more impressive than the genuine kindness and strength we're all capable of?

As I grocery shop, the mother with three kids in tow trying to feed her family humbles me. As I drive down the street, the older man who waits patiently in the snow for the bus humbles me. As I leave for work early in the morning, the student who arrives home from a night of studying humbles me. I smile at these strangers to offer my respect and understanding.

We all have something to offer. We all have something to share. We all have something to learn.

November 7th

I am accepting.

I am accepting because I accept myself. I worked hard to be where I am today. And so have you. Not all salads taste like a cupcake (none actually). Not all exercise routines are as tempting as a night on the couch. You are strong because you ate the salad and worked out regardless. You are strong because you keep moving forward. Each day, you turn the page of this book to improve your wellbeing. Accept yourself for the work you've done. Celebrate your doings. Keep striving each day to be healthier and more positive.

I am also accepting because I accept others. Those who are different from me carry strengths I do not have. They make me smarter and powerful. They have strengths I can benefit from and I have valuable strengths for them, too. I'm accepting of love in my life because love is in me. I am a creature of love and I surround myself with light.

Accept yourself for where you are in this moment. Do your best every day. Accept others with compassion and generosity. They do their best, too.

November 8th

I am a positive influence on my community.

Each recycled water bottle, each walk instead of drive, and each donation of canned goods better your community. It betters your wellbeing, also, through actively curating a better planet and a fulfilled community. For me, when I think of my community, I notice that I'm a positive influence by offering help to people shopping for groceries by suggesting healthy and positive choices.

You can better your community by joining a community garden. You become a part of a group that's hoping to improve the health of others, and it all starts with a pack of seeds.

Right now, think of yourself as a seed in that garden. Others might come and water you, and you might nourish others in return. Soon, you blossom into a plant that has the power to influence health in the lives of your neighbors. When you nourish your community, you cultivate a place of happiness and health for yourself as well.

November 9th

I eat healthful carbs today.

Carbs fill us up and equip us with fuel to power through each day. There are several diets out there that give carbs a bad rep, but we know everything in moderation is good.

Carbs aren't necessarily the snickering enemies that plot your demise over a bubbling cauldron. Carbs can be the wise, consoling idols inspiring you to rule the day, and not let the day rule you. They're the comforting cup of tea on a rainy day. Their true intention is to help you, not burn your tongue or hurt you.

Today pay attention to the carbs you eat and notice the good ones from the bad. Take caution for the ones that cause weight gain, hormone spikes, and inflammation. Determine how many carbs are considered a target for your body type and pay attention to how many you eat today and how you feel. Fruits, rice, pasta, & beans all have carbs. But so do soda, sugar, cakes, and pies. You decide.

Be aware and make your decisions with your eyes wide open. Eat healthy carbs today.

November 10th

I eat only what I need and share what I cannot consume.

There's a feeling of gratification that comes with sharing. The positivity washes over you like sunshine and you are content in that moment.

Today, share what your healthy meals with others. Simply eat what you need. Eat not to fullness, but to that point where you no longer need to eat. Eat to survive *and* to thrive.

Then, knock on your neighbor's door and offer up a casserole dish of your homemade dinner. Ask your co-worker if they'd like a bite of your meal. If you're leaving an extravagant dinner with a box of leftovers in your hand, give your remaining filet mignon to the man looking for food.

Always give to others and give yourself the power of compassion.

November 11th

I take breaks from current events to build up my positive spirit.

Technology provides us with lightning-fast updates on the news all around us. The 24-hour news cycle is right in your hand, the power at your fingertips. Watching current events doesn't always instill hope; whether it's on the news or your preferred platform, sometimes the news of the nation & the world is far too devastating for even the happiest and strong-willed of spirits. This is because we are all essentially connected. Similarly, when a loved one is hurt or broken-hearted, we suffer with them. It's empathy and compassion. It's human nature.

The fork in the road of your wellness journey is that the media mainly focuses on the negative; leaving the positive, courageous, and miraculous segments for puff-pieces rather than breaking news. This leaves us bombarded with negativity, confusion, and worry.

Take breaks from the news. Split your reading into small doses. Be mindful of yourself within this news spectrum. Nurture and keep your spirit elevated. You can do more for you and the world with the right mindset and heart space.

November 12th

Today I bless my back.

Thank you, spine and back, for holding me up every day. I rarely see you, but I do not forget your massive importance. You hold me upright so I can stand and face the day. You provide stability to the rest of my body to protect my soft organs. You are vital to my health. You allow nerves in the spinal cord to travel, sending codes and communicating throughout the body.

I don't need my eyes to know you're there. I scratch you. I pat you. I enjoy those deep massages to feel you in a different way and to soothe you.

When I get upset when you don't feel your best and go out on me, it's not about you. You do a great job. Sometimes you're sick or overworked, just like me when I catch a cold or flu. I'm not mad at you, back. I really just pray for your strength.

Thank you, back, spine, and shoulders. I will treat you well.

November 13th

I use smaller plates to give fuller attention to portion size.

When you attend a dinner party, you automatically fill your plate up; maybe you love your Aunt's scalloped potatoes or your best friend's mac and cheese. We scan for the biggest, heftiest plate and load our vessels with a variety of foods – almost everything that's at the buffet will find its way onto your plate.

But the larger the plate, the larger the portions, and the sooner you start to feel stuffed and uneasy, the kind of fullness where you jokingly plead your spouse to roll you out of the yard like some kind of mutant pumpkin.

Next time you fix yourself lunch or attend a family dinner, try grabbing a smaller plate. Cut back on the excess food you don't need and scoop up the foods you do. Eat until your full. Try smaller portions. Bring awareness to your food. You can enjoy your friend's famous mac & cheese, guilt-free. Truly appreciate the beauty of variety that's found its way onto your plate; try a little bit of everything, simply try smaller portions. Paying attention to your portions is paying attention to your body. Find the balance in your meals.

November 14th

I utilize healthy dinner sharing and sharing with my friends and neighbors for convenience and wellness.

I love a good potluck dinner. Everyone has the opportunity to showcase their chef skills; some bring a cucumber salad or beef stew while others bring a pumpkin pie or homemade ice cream. Sharing meals with friends, neighbors, roommates or extended family makes eating a celebration of love and life. It upgrades your average dinner into a feast of happiness.

Today, tomorrow, or this week, grab your closest friends or loved ones. Organize an evening for a "family dinner." Make it an entertaining challenge, where everyone must bring a vegetable dish or no-added sugars desserts. See what people come up with and even borrow recipes for the future.

If you can, dedicate one day a week to this celebratory dinner. It will become a tradition and each week, you'll look forward to those few hours of chatting and cooking. You come with excitement and leave with leftovers. It's a win-win. Utilize healthy dinner sharing with your nearest and dearest. It's convenient for everyone involved and creates a community of wellbeing.

November 15th

When challenges arise, I ask myself, "what can I learn from this?"

Life is full of ups & downs. It is the universal law of the world. Stop going from zero to 100 every time a challenge arises, running around like the metaphorical chicken with its head cut off. Take a breath. Calm yourself. Look at the issue as an observer looking to positivity and for a happy solution.

Ask yourself, what can I learn from this? In the answer is the solution. The answer will come from within and be about *you*; not your neighbor, or your partner, or your boss who did you wrong.

Once you ask for guidance from your inner self, from the universe, or in your prayers, you will capture your intuition as your answer. Stay open, alert, and positive. God will either change the problem by removing it from your path, or God will leave the problem to change you. For now, build the muscles and strength of character to handle more and more that comes your way with ease and faith.

If you don't hear an answer from your higher power, then the answer is in the question – what can I learn from this?

November 16th

I eat well to have energy for my family.

While we transition into weeks with less sunlight, our days seem to grow longer. Work, approaching holidays, and the hectic pace of life often leave us feeling drained at the end of the day. Yet, it's this transitional season that opens our eyes to our biggest blessing – family.

Family, or the people who love you most, support you and are aware of your dwindling energy. You save up this energy and try to make up on weekends or annual vacations; and even though you might sacrifice your work life or daily schedule, it's worth it to experience the infectious joy brought on through a couple hours of family time.

Remember that you're your own person. It's okay to take a few minutes for yourself during these time-juggling, jam-packed months. Store up your energy for what's important; give your daily best to those who love you and whom you love. Start by eating well for vitality. This will give you clarity to make your best decisions. Choose family. Choose love.

November 17th

I practice kindness.

Be kind to yourself today, before you do anything else. Show compassion for yourself. Repeat in your head throughout the day, "I am a good and worthy person deserving of love and care and tenderness and will cut myself some slack today."

We are products of our upbringing and parenting by nature is infused with guidance. As we mature, we pressure ourselves to live up to a certain expectation or to please others. When we didn't do that, we were considered in our terrible two's or simply rebellious.

Don't put those labels on yourself. You have matriculated, graduated, and come into your own unique being. Be kind to yourself. Show a little self-love. Pat yourself on the back. Give yourself the pep talk you've needed. Don't judge yourself harshly. Find your good qualities and let them shine through your pores like sunbeams. When you are kind to yourself, your kindness will flow to others.

You are a perfect size today. Forget the numbers on the back of your pants. Tear the tag out, if you must. And tomorrow, you will be the perfect size, too. And the next day, and the day after. Give yourself latitude and gratitude to appreciate yourself. It's contagious.

November 18th

I am influencing healthier eating habits for my friends and family.

You woke up this morning. You enjoyed an energizing breakfast. You are widely loved and surrounded by adoration from family and friends. Those family and friends who support you also support your values and ideals. You have a special role that can inspire positivity and wellbeing into your loved ones.

Okay, so you're no personal trainer or nutritionist, but don't discourage yourself; to not include how you've succeeded thus far, through each positive choice, would be a disservice to your effort. You are a vision of health because you have decided to live a life of wellness. By deciding to better yourself, you have accomplished greatness. With each step towards health, you progress towards wellbeing.

You have the power to influence healthier eating habits for your friends and family because you started with your own eating habits. You can be a voice of reason and understanding. Influence those you love with positivity and light.

November 19th

I am flexible, fluid, and ever changing.

Change is inevitable. It's a facet of life that moves you from a curious child to a determined adult. Each day, you're changing; and with these affirmations, you're changing for the better. Avoiding change is to avoid new opportunities for wellbeing. Welcome the transformation. It's a revolution of mind and body and you are leading the riots.

As humans, we learn to adapt to any situation at hand, but we can also challenge the circumstances. Change is inescapable for you on this journey. You will always be moving, growing, and modifying. Don't fear change and don't stand still. Change is growth. Alter your perspective so that a healthy lifestyle is continuously on your mind. Think about the little alterations you can follow through each day. Adapt to your new mindset and go with the ever-changing flow.

November 20th

I am eating slowly today to enjoy my food more.

Take your time today. Proceed through your day with patience. Drift along and observe the chaotic rush people gravitate towards. We constantly rush. From the second we wake up, it's a race to complete our tasks. We speed to meetings, jump over puddles like an obstacle course, and inhale our meals. Especially for lunch breaks during the workday, we rush through our salads and sandwiches to hopefully have a spare minute.

Today, try eating slowly to enjoy your food more. When you slow this process, you gain gratitude for the meal itself. Focus on the tastes, textures, colors, and flavors. Meals shouldn't be scurried through and slammed down, but enjoyed. Ever notice how nauseous you feel after you fly through a meal? Do your body a favor and eat slowly. Find happiness in your meal today by slowing down and appreciating the meal. Acknowledge the process – the process of cooking, the process of digestion, the process of the meal. Turn eating from a physical process to a mental process. Life is not a sprint; it's a marathon. Eat slowly today. Your stomach will thank you.

November 21st

I am inspired by my positive relationships.

Today I will examine my friendships and my family ties by recognizing those who inspire me. I will think about the endless list of characteristics that excite me, and what these people in my life have in common, connected by love, their souls radiating laughter. I will send each of them a silent blessing and reach out with a kind word when I can.

Having the support from someone you admire can make a huge impact on your confidence in yourself and ability to accomplish your dreams and overcome any obstacles in your way. When you see others act and achieve in a way you strive for, it lets you know you have the opportunity to triumph, that you can do it, too. Find out their story. The path to success is paved with failures. Spend time with them, ask them to encourage you - I bet they will give it freely. That's how positive people are. Happiness is contagious.

November 22nd

I am thankful.

Is there someone in your life you've been itching to see? Someone whose schedule rarely matches up with yours, and no matter the time spent apart, you immediately retreat back to that irreplaceable friendship? I met up with an acquaintance the other day who I had lost touch with for over a year.

I'm awe-stricken by how much changes in a year's time. We gabbed about our significant others, our children, and our futures. Taking up a table on a sun-drenched patio, we reclaimed our friendship with no end time constraints, easing through one story to the next. This ability to set aside hours to reminisce and revive relationships provides you an appreciation of life's melody.

Take precious time to be thankful. Look back and pull out the positives. Things could be worse, but they can always become awesomely better. Your perspective shapes your life. The most basic, fundamental foundation for wellness and happiness is recognizing your good fortune. Be thankful. Count your blessings - if you can even count that high.

November 23rd

I am happy to share my meals with other families

Do you ever throw away food? Sometimes you don't clean your plate and discard of the scraps. Sometimes you don't eat the leftovers in the fridge. Sometimes, maybe even every week, you are throwing away food from your fridge that's grown old before you even have a chance to cook it.

There are families who wake up and go to bed hungry. There are landfills of toxic gases growing from rotting products. But there are also solutions that fit nicely with improving your wellbeing and being of service. It's simple. You learned it as a child. It's called sharing.

Find a way to share what you have with others before it hits the garbage can. There are apps and services that facilitate this. Help yourself help others and improve wellbeing for all.

November 24th

I eat well because it nourishes me.

When I eat well, I feel good about myself. I feel like I have accomplished some small feat. I'm satisfied with my meal and my choices, and therefore satisfied with myself. Not necessarily immediately after the meal. But after a week of clean eating? I'm dancing with happiness and I'm glowing with gratitude. Sometimes our body is used to overeating through high-fats or an overdose of sugars. When we decide to eat healthily, our body thanks us from the inside out. Don't be fooled by that mind of yours, the one who sees the commercial for French fries or persuades you to give in to that midnight chocolate craving.

Give more attention to your body. Are you still hungry in your stomach? Or are you allowing emotions to overrun your decisions? Do you feel energized and awake or are you starting to sink into that lazy, lethargic feeling? Choose vitality. Eating well nourishes the body and washes it from the inside out with vitamins and minerals to give you perfect health. How long do you refrain from taking a shower? A day? A week? I don't think so. Now, how long do you avoid a clean diet? Give love to the inside, too. It could use a good wash.

November 25th

My outlook filters what I see.

When you wake up on the wrong side of the bed, the whole day is thrown off. If you're in a bad mood, everything seems to go wrong because you search for the ways it could go wrong. And boy, what an imagination you have. You spill your coffee on your lap during that bumpy morning commute, you forget your lunch at home, you forgot your notes for the big meeting – whatever excuse you can pull out of thin air becomes another building block in your castle of doom. Well, consider me your bulldozer.

Rather than look for the negativity in your life, look for the positivity. Yeah, you spilled your coffee, but how kind was the stranger who offered you a napkin? So you forgot your lunch. Save it for dinner and treat yourself to a healthy afternoon out with friends.

Your outlook filters what you see. Slide on a pair of rose-colored glasses for once. See the world a little better than before. Coax positivity into your life by seeing positivity.

November 26th

Today I make someone else's day better by acknowledging them.

It's been said that all anyone really wants in this life is Appreciation, Affection, and Acknowledgement.

Don't those three A's make you happy? We know that happiness is contagious and, moreover, by the Law of Attraction, we receive what we put out in the world. Acknowledge someone today. It's in your own self-interest.

When you are positive and uplifted, you are in the best mindset to make healthy choices for your life and your body. Doing good makes you feel good, leading to positive choices and before you know it, you're overjoyed. And that's simply by acknowledging others around you. When you acknowledge others, they'll acknowledge you back, and without even noticing, you've added more support to your system.

Share your smile with the world. Acknowledge the positivity that which surrounds you and the many faces it lives behind. Do yourself a favor a make someone else's day better. Oh, the paradox that is shared happiness.

November 27th

I use sauces and dressings sparingly.

Autonomy from enhancements is healthful. The burst of flavor from a fresh tomato stands alone. Calories disguise themselves in creamy dressings and heavy sauces, only to bury the natural taste sensations you strive to enjoy. With the pour of a thick dressing, you destroy the nutritional value of your fruits & vegetables and obliterate their fresh essence. What is originally a healthy meal morphs itself into a health hazard.

Ingredients like salt and sugar camouflage themselves in the opaque sauce. Stay out of the salad dressing aisle and take a detour to the fresh herbs and produce to combine vegetables with a light vinaigrette.

Homemade sauces and dressings made up of natural ingredients, and used sparingly will plate up an enjoyable dining experience. Use your homemade dressings as an accent, not as a base. Fresh ingredients combined in small quantities, like balsamic vinegar with a touch of lemon, add just the right amount of zing to bring out the flavor in any food. Sauces and dressings are whimsical add-ons; don't allow them to become the main dish.

November 28th

Today I will slow down enough to let peace catch up with me and protect me from choices made under stress.

There's a different air when it turns fall. The leaves transform from a forest green to a sunny orange. The slightly chilled wind whisks the fallen leaves around you, occasionally sticking a leaf in your hair like some breed of Autumn Earth Deity. This wind, moving around you, is refreshing. The swirling of the leaves reminds you just how far you can travel, the birds that ride the air remind you just how high you can fly. You are centered in the moment. You are aware.

Today, slow down. Pause and inhale this autumn breeze. Take in the slight coldness of the air, smell the Earth, and find peace around you. If you slow down enough, you allow peace to catch up with you. That peace protects you from the stress and worry in your life. It grants you a moment of solitude to find stillness in your schedule.

Find the calm in each day, but especially today. Observe this changing season. Discover the peace within your own changes. Like the seasons of the year, you are fluid and always evolving. Like the seasons, you are alive.

November 29th

I choose mental satisfaction over physical satisfaction.

The word satiety feels good to me. Once I understood what it meant, it was like a warm blanket encircling me. Fulfilled, satisfied, *spent*. That feeling of euphoric content, moments after you finish your favorite meal or spend time outside doing what you like in perfect weather. Satiety is joy.

Most people are slaves to their physical desire because they are typically quick and don't take much training or effort to get what they want. I'm talking about drinking, drugs, sex, or eating the fatty fried food; the temporary fixes that often leave you mentally exhausted, guilt-ridden and confused.

Choose your mind satiety over flesh satiety. It lasts longer and gives the type of pleasure that is ethereal, heavenly, and lovely. It's a rare breed of satiety, whose effects leave no room for guilt, stress, or regrets. When a physical temptation taunts you, let your mind and your choices for wellbeing control your decision making. You'll become physically satisfied in the long run.

November 30th

I am better every day.

I improve each day. On the days where I'm cruising down the path of wellness, I create positive choices. I distinguish what choices uplift me and continue making those decisions. On the days where I fall off track, I learn from my mistakes. I order the burger, fries, and cherry-topped-milkshake and I observe how it makes me feel. If I'm low-energy or moody, I note to slow down in the speedy drive-thru.

Whether you're having a positive day or a negative day, you are bettering yourself. Not necessarily from the bag of chips or box of chocolates, but learning how these decisions affect you. You learn from your mistakes *and* your wins. You gain a knowledge that sticks with you forever, even on the days where you mess up. You continuously learn and improve each day.

"Success is not final, failure is not fatal: it is the courage to continue that counts." - Winston Churchill

Winter.

December 1st

I am blessed.

There is a higher power always at work for your good. Life is for you. Roadblocks, dreadful conditions, & hurtful people descend upon your journey to strengthen you. Interpret each challenge in your life & ask yourself and your higher power, "What am I supposed to learn from this?"

You learn gratitude. You learn patience. You learn how you are blessed. You are blessed in the good times and the bad, in your coming and your going. You have to open your eyes to see this. If you don't, you'll constantly be fighting the darkness. Don't miss your blessings. Be aware of how unbelievably lucky you are in this life.

Lift your head out of the ground, dust the dirt (or snow) off, and despite the clouds, let the sunshine warm your skin. Happy people aren't happy by accident, or any more blessed than you are. They own their life and their perspective. Once you master it, the Law of Attraction closes in and soon your cup overflows. You are blessed.

December 2nd

I have positive relationships that support my wellbeing.

There is a saying along the lines of, "you are like the top five people you associate with"; it's been attributable to many, so I can't pinpoint who said it first, but people keep repeating it and it rings true. If you hang out with smart, caring, positive people, you will grow in that direction, like a flower that sits on your windowsill in the winter time, leaning towards the warmth of the sunlight through the frosted glass.

Likewise, if you hang around those who are consumed with drama, drinking, & eating excessively (and can't rid themselves of the glass-half-empty neutrality), then that will rub off on you, too. This is self-sabotage. It is difficult to distance yourself from your loved ones, but move them down from the top five to six, to 10, or to 15. Search for those who accomplish projects you want to be a part of and who have been where you want to go. It's like gravity – people have a pull. Give your energy to those that feed your wellbeing and you will feed theirs.

December 3rd

I eat homemade food more than I eat out.

Remember eating around the kitchen or dining room with your family? The food was made fresh, right in front of you. The house smelled great and sounds of laughter would bounce off the walls. As you descended the stairwell, nose guiding your way, mouth-watering, you asked your mom the infamous question, "What's for dinner?"

Our culture has moved away from that tradition. Smartphone features inform you on new restaurant openings, your mail carrier drops off delivery deals, and coupons for free desserts are available at your convenience. But you don't have to follow the crowds. Reclaim the wholeness and goodness of food as well as the love and compassion of eating with family.

Especially around this holiday season, organize a family dinner and opt out of restaurant reservations. What is more satisfying than creating memories around cooking, baking, and eating? Do it once a week. Watch your health as you scratch-make recipes and skip over the preservatives. Eat homemade. It is an important ingredient to your wellbeing.

December 4th

I understand that nothing is certain, and so my faith grows.

Certainty is a myth. Infinite possibilities survive, expanding their availability based on the variety of choices people can make. Some universal laws are true and certain, yet others lack stability at the same time. While it is true the sun will rise tomorrow, there is no guarantee that you will see it. The forecast could predict thunderstorms or Mother Nature could coat the sky in a veil of clouds. An asteroid could hit the earth this afternoon, obliterating it. You can never know for certain what will happen to you, but you can hold faith for tomorrow.

My intention is not to fear monger you into having hope. Quite the opposite. When you recognize nothing is truly certain, that everything changes, ebbs, and flows, then you can release your fear and practice your faith. When you eat right and raise your positive vibrations, you can have faith in a positive outcome. You can't be certain of the when or where, but happier times are ahead when you have faith.

December 5th

I give thanks for each meal before I eat it.

Food is power. Food has the power to change our moods. Its transformational effect can promise a day of crossing off to-do lists, kicking the day's butt with balanced meals and smart snacking. Before you dig into the next meal, feast in the preciously peaceful moment and take a minute to thank your meal.

Look at your food. Consider the beauty of patience & evolution that took milk to convert to cheese. Dedicate a little shout out to the farmers that diligently cared for your cucumbers, spinach, and onions. Show a little gratitude for your food. Where it came from, who took part in its creation, and the distance it's traveled to wind up on your plate.

Give thanks for the meal in front of you, for providing the opportunity to nourish your body with ingredients that will sustain you for years to come, for fueling you through your busy afternoon - for being able to even *have* food. Powerful stuff, right?

You are blessed with opportunity and miracles. Rejoice.

December 6th

I wait 5 minutes before I satisfy a craving for fast food to give myself time to make the best choice for me.

In the past, cheeseburgers and fries were luxuries. They were a treat, a sign of celebration. Now, our avenues are lined with fast food options, from double-deckers on demand to a tour of Tex-Mex. We're also bombarded with advertising for these unhealthier options. We carry miniature billboards in our hands, otherwise known as smart phones, that send us updates on the latest in the fast food empire. With cheap prices and images of options at our fingertips, it's no wonder we frequent fast food more than any country in the world – it's everywhere.

Today, instead of running to your nearest drive-thru after seeing an enticing commercial, wait 5 minutes before you grab your keys. Wait five minutes before you indulge in fast food to provide yourself the time to consider your craving and make the best choice for yourself. Don't be a victim to the advertising game. Be your own advertisement: an endorsement of health.

December 7th

Today I bless and appreciate my stomach that does a wonderful job digesting the food I put in it.

Your stomach is strong. It's flexible. It reflects each choice you make through action. It can be bloated at times and slow you from squeezing into that old pair of jeans, or you could wake up one morning to find your tummy flattened.

Beneath your surface skin, your stomach is working to turn your food choices into movement and action. Your stomach shoots off warning signs to let you know when you're full or when you're hungry. Your stomach works with your mind to find the right choices that work for your body and your energy. Through your stomach, those healthy choices create a healthy chain of reaction by absorbing nutrients and spreading them throughout your system. It starts with your mind, yes, but your stomach is next in line.

Listen to it – the gurgling sounds after a fatty meal signal it's a bit too much on that stomach of yours. But the peaceful sound of digestion shows you're doing something right. Pat your tummy today. Let that stomach know you appreciate all it does for you.

I will drink a tall glass of water before I have a second helping of food.

Water is a great cleanser. It washes away the old to bring in the new and ushering in a fresh new start. Like a cold shower or hot, bubbly bath. Why do you think it's so thrilling to chill out by the beach or swimming pool?

Use water and all of its refreshing and healing properties to assist you in your journey to wellness. Typically, one serving of food is more than enough for our bodies to function well (especially with America-sized portions). A second helping is for taste or to fill an emptiness.

It would be great to fill the emptiness with a thought of awareness for why or what you are avoiding. However, when you don't want to take time for self-reflection in the middle of the party, just have a glass of water first. Let it do the work of cleaning for you.

"Nothing is softer or more flexible than water, yet nothing can resist it." – Lao Tzu

December 9th

I practice compassion.

Everything is a practice. You don't speak well with your first sentence or walk long distances with your first steps. The more diligently you focus on each task, the better you become at it. Today, I decide to practice compassion.

Compassion is like giving an emotional hug to everyone you meet. Imagine that. Once when exploring my way through a town in Oregon with a friend, she mentioned there were people who were giving away free hugs in the busy city center. Hugs, for free. I thought it was odd and slightly cute at the same time. Now, I understand it. They were physically manifesting compassion.

You don't have to organize a free-hug fundraiser, but you can open your heart to send love and you can vision giving someone a hug. It can be a little uncomfortable at first. It takes practice. Start by being compassionate towards yourself. Then with your family or your spouse (especially when they are in a bad mood), and move onto coworkers and strangers. Now that's good practice.

December 10th

I believe and declare I am everything God created me to be.

There are some things science doesn't fully explain. Coincidence has no hypothesis. Miracles are not a theory. Some things just happen with no black or white explanation.

There are those moments where we are unsure of a higher power or God's presence. I searched for answers when I wanted to leave my corporate career but didn't know how. But I realized that I worked through those challenges for a reason. Each struggle makes me stronger. God gave me those struggles to thicken my skin and amplify my voice.

If you don't believe there's a God or a higher power, believe that the universe has come together to bring you exactly where you are. You are not a mere coincidence. You are purposeful. Believe that you are everything your higher power created you to be. You are the rare flower that blooms between the cracks of the cold concrete sidewalk. Marvel at yourself; you are a wonder. The more you recognize this, the more you add to your healthy, happy existence.

December 11th

Today I focus on protein.

Focus on protein today that nourishes the ecosystem as much as it nourishes your body. Plant-based proteins such as edamame, black beans, or oatmeal fill you up while powering you through those long work days and busy afternoons.

Protein is all around you. Don't pigeonhole it to steak and eggs. Unveil the unknown homes of protein. Challenge yourself to replace your *beef bourguignon* with an Asian-inspired tofu. Tofu in itself absorbs any flavor in the pantry; easy to cook, and on your digestive system, it's an adaptable protein that could be used from tacos to main dishes.

What were once protein replacements have taken center stage as the lead role. Broccoli, spinach, and avocado hold the nutritional talent to satisfy while improving your health. A handful of almonds can steer you from that 3 o'clock slump and curb your cravings for that bag of chips. And with the endless ways to prepare these options, you could fill each day of the week with a fresh thought for dinner. Try something new. Make eating a fabulous adventure.

December 12th

The scale only has the power that I give it to change my mood.

When you rely on outside sources, people, or measures to determine your mood, you give away your power. Each of us is powerful. We are created that way. It is our default position. The only variable is, do we give our power away, leave it dormant through inertia, or do we live up to our full potential?

I am certainly guilty of stepping on the scale and just being disgusted. Then, I'm in an unpleasant mood. I reinforce that mood by calling up friends or giving myself a critical once-over in the mirror. Take your power back. If you must weigh yourself on the scale, limit it to the same time and day of the week. Otherwise, use cues to gauge your wellbeing, not your quantity of mass. Check in with yourself. How do you feel? Is it a 3-star or 5-star day? Is your energy aligned with what you want to accomplish? Eat for those feelings. Find your power and positivity.

December 13th

I substitute positive activities for my nighttime habit of snacking.

Winding down after the day is one of my favorite times. Like a sigh of relief, you sip some chamomile tea and relax into the evening. The day has past and with a sufficient night's sleep, you'll be able to take on another vivacious 24 hours.

But, it can be difficult to fight the urge to snack. In between that period of post-dinner and pre-sleep and you want something to send you off to your cozy bed. My friend's excuse is that she eats dark chocolate and it's filled with antioxidants. Even so, that evening chocolate craving has developed into a nighttime habit of snacking. We all have a nightly ritual that signals it's time for bed, and I know she's not the only one who sniffs out the sugar hiding in the cupboards.

This evening, try a different approach to rounding out the night. Read a chapter of a book. Meditate to ease your mind. Journal to reflect on your afternoon. Do something besides scouring the pantry. Notice how you sleep better. Take in that energetic feeling for the next morning. Substitute positive activities for your nighttime snacking.

December 14th

I am generous.

Generosity is cyclical; when you devote kindness and charity towards others, kindness returns in your favor. Qualities like thoughtfulness, selflessness, and grace connects us to others, creating friendships with once-strangers.

How does generosity improve your health? It could be physical, like running a marathon to raise funds for those suffering from terminal illnesses. It could be mental, like organizing toiletry kits for the homeless. It could be emotional, like listening to your friend's woes after a stressful day. Wellness and health doesn't stop at the scale, it's a learning process towards a healthier you, to become a better version of yourself. The version you're working to become. Attract positivity with generosity.

Give. Be generous. Donate money and time to better your community and, eventually, the world. Give to others and you will give to yourself. Do good; it makes you feel great.

December 15th

This week, I will have salad at least one meal per day.

During the chillier winter months, we choose comfort foods over fresher options. Soup, pasta, and chili thrive in this season. It's when the snow hides the grass that we overlook the magical healing powers of fresh produce.

Salads are delicious; luscious lettuce topped with crisp cucumbers, the softness of tomato slices which offset the earthiness of carrots. If you replace one meal a day with one antioxidant-wielding salad, it will improve your mood and your body. Rather than thick dressings or cheese, choose a light vinaigrette or creamy avocado.

This type of eating well will leave you energetic, not groggy and lethargic. You may even find that the necessary fiber moves your metabolism and keeps you happily regular.

Some people think it's a waste of a good meal to just eat a salad. I say it's uplifting to eat a meal that leaves you buoyant and feeling good about your willpower and determination. One change per day makes a big difference. Watch it add up.

December 16th

I understand that only light can dissolve darkness.

Hate does not discount hate, only love can win. Love always wins. As overused as that statement is, it's infamous because it's accurate. The only thing stronger than darkness is light. Light obliterates the shadows; it beams through whatever is in its path.

Sometimes when I'm upset, I'll call a dear friend of mine who is guaranteed to make me laugh. With sarcasm and an R-rated pun here and there, she'll find the joke somewhere. Her wisecracking lightheartedness becomes light. When you're down and a friend makes you laugh, it's an instant mood changer. Thank God for the people in your life who have a loaded gun of one-liners and a passion to make you laugh. Personify their hilarious mindset so you can bring light into your life. Illustrate a fresh perspective on finding the hidden good, which always lies in the perceived bad. Laughter overruns tears.

Find the light and you will no longer be cast in the shadows. Discover happiness through each sliver of sunshine. Wake up and let the light in. Illuminate your soul.

December 17th

I have constant access to healthy foods to increase my wellness.

Make sure you keep things handy for when you need them. Do you have a certain place in your home or car for your wallet or your keys or cell phone? Imagine not having easy access to these items, especially if you're in a rush. Most of us have placed a level of priority on being connected and experience a sense of loss or disconnectedness when that cell phone is broken or misplaced.

Your health is astoundingly more important than almost anything else, yet we don't keep access to healthy food as a priority. Change that today. Just like reaching for your cell phone, quickly reach for fruits, seeds, veggies, and nuts. Keep a bottle of water within arm's reach.

Make constant access to healthy snacks a priority. Invest in your health with the same priority of grabbing your keys before you lock the door.

December 18th

I talk on the phone after I eat.

It can be relaxing to fix a dinner, sit down, and to phone a friend. If you're lucky enough to chat on video, it's like having dinner together. You're sharing a meal with a loved one. This is nice occasionally. To do it regularly, however, robs you of that rare alone time to focus on your wellbeing.

Eating is a cherished and important part of your health and wellbeing. It's meant to be a time where you connect with the dish itself. You take in the flavors and textures, swallowing each bite with care. This experience is diluted if you are the phone while you're eating. You split your attention.

Of course, sometimes you're terribly busy where you must eat while dialing phone numbers or multi-tasking. Yet, if this is your norm, you actively dismiss your wellbeing to the back seat. Check your priorities. Eat - then talk. And when you eat, *eat*.

December 19th

I am happy to benefit from foods my friends share with me.

We have friends and family over fairly regularly and we look forward to sending them home with an extra plate of food for the rest of the family. We also enjoy when they share with us. That's one less lunch I have to pack or dinner I have to make.

I am blessed with new flavors and foods that I may not be familiar with, thanks to these friends and family of mine. And no two people cook exactly the same. Do you level your measurements or round that teaspoon of sugar? Maybe you just throw in a pinch. The nuances create an experience with friends. Food is very intimate, even for those who take it for granted. Sharing increases your intimacy with others and saves time and waste. It's one of those great blessings. The gift is in the giving and also in the receiving.

December 20th

I recognize that alcohol lowers my resolve to eat healthy.

I'm a wine enthusiast. Over the years, wine has skyrocketed in popularity to become the drink of choice for the masses. It has become socially acceptable to have a comforting glass or two of wine to wind down in the evenings, reflecting on the afternoon while basking in those peaceful nights.

But not everything that glitters is gold; alcohol, as relieving as it may be, dulls your brain. Alcohol alters your decision-making and your response time (hence why you should never drink and drive). If you embark on a journey to happiness through eating well, alcohol will lower your capacity to make the best choices.

Be mindful. While you initially could limit yourself to one drink so you won't snack afterward, one hearty glass of wine can change your mind. Next thing you've thrown up your hands in defeat and the snacking ensues. Promote yourself towards positivity and stay aware, whether eating or drinking.

December 21st

I am aware that sugar contributes to inflammation in my body.

Some say sugar is the new smoking. Others say a sedentary lifestyle is. Either way, we can argue that smoking is bad for your health and it is highly discouraged. Thus, sugar and a sedentary lifestyle are, too.

As a past-smoker, I can say I was blinded by my habit. I thought I was healthy because I ran, worked out, and ate well. Three years after my last puff, I feel how much more open my lungs are and how much smoother my skin feels.

Like smoking, sugar can develop into a habit and an addiction. And that habit can grow to hurt your health, causing fat to accumulate or teeth to rot. While I was in the midst of an unhealthy habit, I couldn't compare my present health to anything else. Since I've quit, I know what wellness feels like. When you skip the sugar in your diet, you start to know what health feels like.

Sugar causes inflammation in your body. In high quantities, it leads to obesity and other health traps. Recognize and reduce your exposure to sugar. Increase your wellbeing.

December 22nd

I am making a conscious choice to avoid caffeine today.

I've given up coffee more times than I can remember. I would read the side effects of caffeine, like insomnia, nervousness, & nausea, and cut it out of my morning routine (and afternoon pit-stop). Cold turkey. Always at three days in, I am relentlessly plagued with a throbbing migraine. I learned that my body was working through withdrawals. It was responding to my lack of coffee, and boy, was she outraged.

Caffeine is addictive. It's okay to have in general and on occasions; sometimes coffee can rev up your metabolism, and it's even been linked to lowering risk of Type 2 diabetes. But mull it over. Think about it. Addictive? Why attach your body to anything that has power over it? For almost every fast or diet, caffeine is always on the "no" list. This journey to wellness is about understanding your own power and taking control of your life to achieve happiness and your purpose. Take control with one thing at a time. Lose your addiction. Make a conscious choice to avoid addictions today.

December 23rd

Gratitude allows me to accentuate my positivity.

My Godmother, who is approaching 80 (I think), recently told me, "I'm fine as wine and right on time!" She said this while fluttering across the kitchen, cooking a traditional Sunday breakfast, filled with love, light, and an amount of butter that could send a professional athlete to heart disease. The food was not the lowest in calories or had the highest nutritional value, but when you have a homemade meal, infused with the love and care that only the bond of family can produce, the benefit for wellbeing outweighs a minor (major?) calorie infraction.

Moreover, in those breakfast table moments with wisdom floating around the room, take time to be thankful for the lessons. She said she never understood why people speak negatively about themselves. The usual repertoire of self-hate: "I'm fat," "I'm old," or "I can't do that." God made each of us different and perfect in our own unique circumstance. When we give thanks and express gratitude for what we do have, we can more easily see and appreciate the gifts we offer this world. So, you go be *Fine and On Time* today – if an 80-year-old can do it, so can you.

December 24th

I choose peace.

You cannot heal what you do not know. You choose to heal based on where you focus your attention. Negative feelings in any form are blaring alarm bells to wake you up to a blockage that holds you back from peace and happiness. These blockages show up as resentment, jealousy, hate, envy, anger and other negative emotions.

It does not matter if you think you are right or someone did you wrong. If you are right, then simply be right. Only you need to know you are right. You do not need to tie yourself in knots trying to convince someone else. Or are you telling yourself a story? Release the burdens. These negative minds perpetuate bad habits like overeating and self-medicating, dulling your sense of indignation.

When you focus on why you have the negative emotion, you can choose to free yourself. A peace will wash over you and your best choices for your life will come to you. Choose awareness. Choose happiness. Choose peace.

December 25th

Gratitude allows me to harness the positive energy I need to receive grace.

Being grateful opens up your gates and barriers to receive all the goodness life has to offer you. It's like opening your door during the holiday season to welcome friends bearing gifts, presents wrapped with metallic wrapping paper, glitter-covered ribbon, and tags saying your name. You look around your cozy living room, grasp your cup of hot cocoa, and are truly content with life at that present moment.

On the contrary, when there are no thanks, the door stays closed, the wrapping paper nowhere to be found, your carpet glitter-less. You wonder if you are making progress. Begin each day by giving thanks to anything and everything. Begin each meal by taking a moment to say thank you for the nourishment. Bring this into your daily life - your happiness will flourish and you will easily achieve more of your heart's desires.

"Wear gratitude like a cloak and it will feed every corner of your life." -Rumi

December 26th

I am eating for my wellbeing more and eating out of habit less.

It takes 21 days to make a habit. Most of us have grown accustomed to eating habits formed over lifetimes. We learn by example from parents, peers, and the media, telling us when to eat and what to crave. Indulging in cravings or emotional eating are strong habits to kick, but instead of focusing on ending old habits, challenge yourself to focus on building new habits.

Today, eat for your wellbeing. Make mindful eating your new habit. Mindful eating is paying attention and considering your eating routine through how it affects your body, mind, and spirit. Notice how different foods produce different moods. How does your productivity change when you nourish your body with clean nutrition? Do you gain positivity or peace of mind? Follow those feelings. Chase them with each bite of a juicy strawberry, a savory quinoa salad, or a hummus scooped cucumber. Eat not because you're feeling blasé or sad, but eat because your body craves nutrition. Today, eat because you need, not because you want.

December 27th

I have joy.

Joy is a feeling of inner happiness. It does not pass by and is not fleeting. Happiness may come and go depending on your circumstance, but joy is constant and continuous. We all have joy. I have it and you have it, even when you're low or not your best. Joy is inherent in our makeup. It's like having blood or skin. It's that fundamental. We only need to access it and harness it.

If you knew there was an account at a random bank in Utah with $7 million waiting for you, how hard would you try to access it? The deeper question is, do you consider yourself rich, even before you find it? This is how joy is. It is a deep knowing that all is well. No matter what comes and goes, all is well.

Peel back the layers covering your access to joy. Work at it like you are searching for your treasure. It's there. Within you. Joy.

December 28th

I walk up stairs more every day.

When you're rushing to your desk or carrying armfuls of groceries, the elevator is usually chosen over the stairwell. Why struggle and sweat when you can peacefully glide up the building? Those beads of sweat mean you're working hard. It signals a dedication to your metabolism and muscles. It's a dedication to your wellbeing.

Simply adding more stairs to your daily movement can alter your activity levels and your energy. The flight of stairs makes the ultimate difference in your health and our culture's sedentary lifestyle. It's those extra steps today that can be a whole stairwell next week.

Don't push yourself to walk hundreds of stairs, but actively ascend the stairwell a small amount each day. Know that with each step, you're climbing towards progress. You'll get there if you continuously do your best each day. Take it one step at a time (literally).

December 29th

I am eating only fruits and vegetables today.

If you walk into the grocery store, you're instantly met with a variety of processed foods. They might greet you as you walk in to let you know there's a sale, so take advantage of the three-bags-for-$4 deal. Processed foods overrun our diets; sometimes because they're right in front of our faces. There's a plethora of processed merchandise available, so much so that we often fail to recognize our money-saving conveniences are leaving out space for the healthful foods.

Today, commit to eating foods that are grown and not engineered or processed. Vegetables, rice, beans, and fruits are considered plant based. Frozen dinners, pizza, and sandwiches are not. By taking a processed food vacation, you pay attention to how much manipulated food you eat. The real eye-opener here may be recognizing how unusual it is to not have processed meals throughout the day.

This awareness will move you to change the direction of your eating habits for the better. Take time today to focus on only eating plant-based foods.

December 30th

I express gratitude every day.

Start giving thanks throughout the day. Not just when someone opens the door or passes you the orange juice. Not out of politeness or habit. But out of real, sincere gratitude. A "you didn't have to do it" type of thankfulness. Unexpected, but loved nonetheless.

Who makes the differences in your life? What is something new you're excited about? When you look in the mirror, what excites you? Be thankful. I have a friend who comes and helps me move every time I relocate. She volunteers her time, without me asking like some kind of guardian angel who floats down when I need her golden organizational touch. I'm always appreciative on the days my husband stops his route home to pop into the store and pick up something I might like for dinner. And how could I forget the times my daughter calls me for no reason other than to say hello? Let gratitude encompass you. These shoes are comfortable, hugging my ankles without cramping my toes. My rings feel a little looser today. My mom is feeling well this week.

From big to small, express thanks. It raises your energy to receive even more blessings and to be a blessing to others.

December 31st

My goals align with my spirit.

When your goals are aligned with your spirit, you are aligned to the universe. Imagine the many different ways you can make micro-shifts within yourself to ease your journey to wellbeing.

Your personality fits with your endeavor. Your pathway is right for your type of driving. Do you like highways or dirt roads? City driving or scenic routes? Where is your music volume set? Do you need to slow it down or is it too low you need to crank it up?

The people in your circle understand you and are a part of your endeavors. Do they laugh at your jokes and support your vision? Do they respectfully challenge you to be better and help make your dreams and reality?

Your talents are able to be seen. Do you have hidden talents? That's the shame. Let them out. Your spirit wants to unleash its purpose through your talents.

What is in your spirit? Let it out. Then, set your goals accordingly.

January 1st

I am motivated.

What motivates you? What is your purpose? Answering this fundamental question launches you towards a path to happiness and wellbeing. A basic question, but most people refuse to take the time to reveal what their divine potential is. This knowledge is essential. If you don't know where you are going, you'll end up anywhere; a map is useless if you don't know where you are and where you want to be.

Find your motivation. Follow this:

1. Close your eyes.

2. Ask yourself what is my purpose?

3. Take 3 deep breaths and remain quiet.

4. When you open your eyes think about what your intuition is telling you.

Listen to your gut. Your inner voice already knows what you're called to do. When you eliminate the white noise, you can hear it smoothly whispering to you. Reiterate your purpose daily. There will be shifts based on circumstance, but what motivates you is a gift in your core, waiting to be unwrapped. Open it today.

January 2nd

I find my true self in stillness.

When you are busy and have a million thoughts running through your mind, you miss the ability to see your fullest potential. People believe that busy work and filling every minute of the day is living up to their fullest potential. This tends to be exactly wrong. It is filling the time throughout the day with activity. You recognize your fullest potential by taking time in the quiet and stillness to hear and know in your soul what your next best steps are.

Imagine living in a mansion, but you only stay in one room or even one wing, cleaning and fiddling in the same rooms day after day. You miss all that the rest of the house has to offer - the media room, a craft room for your artistic expression, a library of your favorite types of books. Be still. Find your true self.

"Why do you stay in prison, when the door is wide open?" – Rumi

January 3rd

Eating well makes me feel good about my choices.

Choose health and wellness for one month. Notice how you feel today. What would you like to improve? Is your skin showing the signs of stress? Do you want that pain in your leg to subside? A desire for the backaches to end? Along with the bloating and secret gas? (Don't blame it on the dog; he had nothing to do with you picking up that mac & cheese on your route home.)

When you choose to eat well for your health, your life will improve in infinite ways. This does not mean you need to go on a fad diet. Throw the crash diets out of your mind. Rather, adjust your current diet with conscious decisions and food choices that improve your condition. Stop eating thoughtlessly. Your food is important and needs attention, more so than the outfit you wear tomorrow or the plans you have for the weekend. Live your best life now. Choose to eat well.

January 4th

I practice in the present what I am doing in the future.

We want everything now. Our streets are lined with fast food options, our technology delivers us information immediately, and companies have employed shortcuts in production for quick profits. We also have a culture that is increasingly depressed, on medication, and sick. We can't keep up with this manufactured pace, and sacrifice our sanity in the name of immediate results. What you do today will manifest in the future, so slow down and pay attention. The tiny mustard seed planted today will soon sprout into a strong trunk and wide branches. An egg fertilized will take nine months to birth a baby. Meat marinated overnight and slow-cooked on a smoker will yield you a tantalizing dish full of flavor.

Take time to do the things today that will yield the beautiful results you want in the future. It won't be instantaneous, but anything worth having is worth waiting for. Be healthy tomorrow, by making healthy choices and eating well today.

January 5th

I can only change what I am aware of.

How can you work on something without knowing what it is you're improving? If your boss approaches you with a task, you know the problem at hand so that you may fix the issue. The same goes for your health – you must know what it is about yourself that you wish to improve so you can improve those characteristics.

Once you pinpoint your problem areas, then you can actively work on them. You must know your goals so you can achieve your goals on this journey. Progress each day at a time and transform your health.

You can only change what you are aware of; if you refuse to admit the areas of weakness, you won't be able to strengthen them. This isn't an opportunity to bash your appearance or complain about your life. It's a positive chance to notice the areas of your life that could use a little tune-up. Do you eat too much meat? Drink too much wine? Don't get enough rest or exercise? Confess it.

What are you aware of today? And how will that affect your journey?

January 6th

I am prepared.

Life seems to run effortlessly when we take time out of our busy mornings or late nights to plan and prepare for our foreseeable futures. We plan for the day – what we will wear and eat, or for the year – what vacation and traveling will we book. Preparation keeps the stress down while readying you to be at your best for the challenges or constraints that confront you.

My husband is a chef so he always talks about his *mise en place* (pronounced meez-ahn-plahs). It's a French culinary term meaning everything in its place. To me, it means he's organizing all of his ingredients together so when he starts cooking, he's prepared for each step with the recipe at his fingertips. With every clove of garlic, sprig of thyme, or dash of pepper, he's prepared.

You can practice your own version of *mise en place* for a healthy diet and a vivacious life. Control what you can each day with preparation. You'll find yourself surrounded by abounding opportunities. Your charmed and healthy life is waiting for you right around the corner.

"Luck is what happens when preparation meets opportunity." -Seneca the Younger

January 7th

My spiritual true self and my worldly self are congruent.

Sometimes when you're curating your passion or working on a project that excites you, you're overcome with this spark of higher power. Regardless of what action you're doing, when you do what you love, that tiny speck of light inside you shines to grasp your attention. Take the flickering flame and grow it into a wildfire.

When you follow your passion, you're following your purpose. Even if you're not particularly good at it, keep going. Practice every day. The light you feel is your spiritual self-breathing life into your worldly self - you are connecting your soul with mind and body. It's beyond magical; it's otherworldly.

Every day, search for the ways to find that spark again. Breathe and know that it's in you. It's in everyone, but not everyone has the courage to throw propane on the match. Be brave and pursue your passion. Match up your true self and bring the light back into your body.

January 8th

I will subscribe to a wellness blog.

It takes awareness and attention of a goal to achieve it. Living a healthier lifestyle is not about counting calories; it's immersing in the conversation. It's becoming a part of something bigger than yourself and contributing, if only with your presence.

Do something today to deepen and further your understanding and commitment to living a healthier life. Subscribe to a blog or two. There is a world of interesting content available to you – and it's free. Devote an hour to a regular publication, blog, or site you can join.

Don't know where to start? Sit quietly for a minute. Close your eyes and take a few deep breaths. Start with the *UGottaEat* blog or your preferred search engine. Trust that when you seek, you will find.

"Day by day, what you choose, what you think, and what you do is who you become." – Heraclitus

January 9th

When I am bored, I find productive ways to fill that void and maintain healthy eating habits.

We are blessed to live in an age where opportunity is at our fingertips. There are thousands of activities you could be doing right this second – volunteering at a shelter, reading that dust-covered book, signing up for a scuba diving class.

But, instead of challenging ourselves, we head to the kitchen pantry to pass the time. Boredom snacking develops a habit of eating when you're not hungry. You eat because it's something to do, it supplements your nightly cable binge, or it's another stop on that long road trip.

Rather than exploring your refrigerator for the hundredth time, explore your surroundings. Rediscover your interest in an old talent. Practice yoga. Call a friend across the country simply to say hi. Find productive ways to fill the void of the boredom black hole. Stay on track towards your goal of health.

January 10th

I am disciplined.

Speak what you want into existence. If you want even more of it, write it down. And if you really, honestly want it, practice it daily. Whatever it is. Today you can start with a very practical and foundational affirmation of top of which so many desires can be achieved.

You are disciplined. You do what you say and say what you do. Not just one time, but over and over again you make a commitment and you keep it. You are honest this way. And trustworthy. And loyal. Not just to other people, but to you. It's most important that you can rely on you. You are your best ally.

If you hear people say, "I'm my own worst enemy," send them a blessing because they are working against themselves. Don't do that to yourself. Lift yourself and accomplish your goals. You are awesome. You are disciplined.

January 11th

I eat only 1 serving which is enough to nourish me.

In the past, I would scoff at the serving size suggestion printed on nutrition facts. "Meant for two people," became a challenge rather than a suggestion. I'm sure we've all done the same - ate more servings than needed, dropping our forks in defeat.

Today, recognize how many servings you truly ingest. Eat only one serving for each meal. That one serving, while it may look initially small, is all you need for nourishment. The only reason it looks minuscule is because we've overshot our serving sizes. Everything is super-sized or doubled. Rewire your brain to recognize the size of the servings you truly need. You've been trained through witty advertising to think otherwise.

If you're out to dinner, don't eat everything on the plate. Try and box up leftovers. Take the rest home to share with your family members or roommates. Know how much your body needs by following the serving size recommended on those nutrition labels. Observe how you feel afterward.

January 12th

I remind myself that others have the same issues that I do.

Everyone struggles. You could be a part of a tribe in an indigenous country or a CEO of an international company, and you still would worry about working, about your family, or why you haven't been asked out to dinner.

Why do we struggle? We try to prove to others how hard we have it, how our problems are bigger than theirs. This is a losing game where no one wins.

Obstacles are normal. Remember that your problems do not overshadow the problems of others. Next time someone confides in you about their difficulties listen before responding with your own rebuttal. Rather than enter into a complaining competition, show support for others as they encounter troubles. Release your ego and create an atmosphere of endearment and love. Allow positivity to overflow your life in all aspects imaginable.

January 13th

Success is not determined by the brilliance of my plan, but by the consistency of my actions.

No one knows what they are doing. Honestly. Do you think Bill Gates (or any other millionaire tech guru) had a master plan after dropping out of college? They didn't. But, they knew what they wanted to do. They acted and along the way learned how to accomplish their wildest dreams.

We exhaust ourselves in preparation to the point where we are far too spent to follow through with our agendas. Simplify the process. Remind yourself every day of your goals. Think about your desired future before you act. Then, act.

Success generates not from a to-do list, but from your actions. Learn from personal experience how to accomplish your goals; that wisdom is only unveiled if you start working. Take the risk to act. Once you jump that leap of faith, change will transform your life. Don't talk the talk, walk the walk. Be a person of action.

January 14th

I am the master of my fate.

Your life starts with you. With each thought, sentence, and action, you determine how your life will proceed. There will always be loved ones who offer golden nuggets of advice, but only you know what you need and want.

Once you know you're the master of your fate, you can decide to take control of your destiny. Then, the universe and your higher power will work with you to transport you to success. The universe helps those who are actively helping themselves. You must set a trend of positivity and activity, and the universe will join in on the party.

Acknowledge your own power. You can either choose to stay where you are or choose to create the life you've desired. Only you decide your fate.

"Nothing will work unless you do." – Maya Angelou

January 15th

I pack my lunch the day before.

During these chillier months, I find it more difficult to wake up on time. You're huddled in your blanket cocoon, when you're violently interrupted by the buzzing of an alarm, the starter pistol to a rushed morning.

During these rushed mornings, we forget to pack a lunch. We abandon our meal plan to make it to work or school on time, resorting to take-out.

Avoid the unhealthy temptation of the take-out lunch (and enjoy a few extra minutes of peaceful slumber) by packing your lunch the day before. This small step keeps you headed in the direction of a positive lifestyle. It reduces stress *and* it boosts your energy with nutritious, homemade options. The few minutes to make your lunch the night before will miraculously turn into 10 extra minutes in the morning.

This step might seem small now but just wait until that 6 a.m. alarm rings in your ear. You'll be wishing you did this sooner.

January 16th

I bring loving attention to my skin today.

Feel your skin. Trace over the bumps and the smoothness, study the lines and the coloring. Thank your skin for its cover and protection. Admire it for keeping your body safe from cuts and scrapes. No matter what you have thought about your looks or your skin, recognize right now what an awesome and miraculous function it has in making you, you.

Your skin is a tell-all for your body and health. You might encounter a rash when you come in contact with something harmful or unhealthy. Your skin raises in goosebumps in reaction to a sensation or realization. You laugh when tickled in certain spots. Your pores open up, allowing sweat to regulate your body temperature. Your skin heals itself to keep you safe from disease. Admire your skin for its strength. Pamper your skin for all it's done. Take some Vitamin E. Soothe it with a luxurious moisturizer. Thank you, skin.

January 17th

I am buying healthful foods today in preparation for eating healthy later this week.

You eat what's in your kitchen. If a bag of artificial cheese-dusted puffs is within reach, you can bet that's your first choice. Rather than choose unhealthier options in the moment, choose the healthy options at the store. Prepare in advance for those moments where the bag of chips is your first option by not making them an option at all.

Today, buy healthful foods to prepare for healthier eating – for today, tomorrow, and later in the week. Similarly, to a friend group, who or what you surround yourself with will become a reflection of you. If trans fats or artificial sugars surround you, then your health and mood will reflect those choices. If vegetables and hummus beckon your name, you'll benefit from the vitamins and protein of your positive snack choice.

Choose smartly by buying mindfully. Keep healthy choices handy so those are the choices you gravitate towards.

January 18th

I am courageous.

Everything you need is already within you. The right decisions to that difficult challenge are patiently waiting to be uncovered. But it's there. Many people desperately desire to leave a job they hate, or to speak up for themselves but don't muster the courage to do so. It's tragic to see an unhappy worker become laid-off in a downturn when they could have left on their own accord and found happiness proactively instead of reactively.

Release your bottled-up inner voice. Believe that you are made to be happy. Understand that negative occurrences are your opportunity to exercise courage. Have the courage to apply for other jobs, take a leave of absence, update that resume. Have the courage to make yourself a priority, to restart your energy and recharge your spirit. Square those shoulders and hold your head up high. You have courage within you.

January 19th

I am complete.

You are complete. You are enough. You are divine. Too often we focus on the aspects of ourselves that we don't like. The world has conditioned us that way. But it's okay because today, you can recondition your thinking. You will begin to know deep down inside that your positives outweigh your negatives - and *that* is where you should put your attention.

Imagine a small compact mirror with a crack, splayed throughout its surface. Now imagine a huge wall mirror with the same size crack, hiding off in a corner by the floor. You are the big mirror, perfectly absorbing and reflecting light. The small crack is perfect in its imperfection. It gives you character and personality. Embrace it, but moreover, enjoy the totality of the mirror. You are not a small mirror with a big crack. You are a large beautiful reflection of life with wonderful characteristics that make you, you. You are complete just as you are. Cracks and all.

January 20th

I maximize my metabolism by eating well.

Your metabolism is your weight-loss secret weapon. It works behind the scenes, under layers of skin and flesh to burn calories and transform your meals into energy. The energy that keeps your brain focusing, blood pumping, and your waist tightening. Exercising and eating healthy can help your metabolism work even harder than it already does.

Today, maximize your metabolism through eating well. Drink two liters of water; dehydration can slow metabolism. Opt for green tea, known to burn fat, over coffee for your morning wake up call. Choose lean proteins with iron. Spicy foods like chili peppers jumpstart your metabolic rate, too, thanks to antioxidants. Squeeze in these samples when you can to revive your metabolism. The more energy you have, the more willing you are to continue with positive choices and the more active you become.

January 21st

I get things done when I fixate my full attention on my goal.

Bumps along the road of life are not excuses to veer off course. Take my fateful day of the broken pants zipper: I ate clean for weeks, my skin smooth, and my bowel movements stellar. But when I slipped on those blue jeans, buttons holding on for dear life, I was discouraged. As I considered indulging in a treat day to heal my bruised ego, I realized I am blossoming into wellness, one patient day at a time.

That same afternoon, I was emotionally challenged when I received unfortunate news about a friend who had passed away. My heart was heavy as I was departing another funeral at that same time. Two lives lost, both so close to my heart, in a matter of a week? It was a recipe for diet disaster. Part of me wanted nothing more than to fill the voids in my heart with whatever junk food I could find. Instead, I turned my full attention on my goals to be a healthier, stronger, better person. My friends and loved ones need me, so I need to be at my best. I must support their lives with love and light as best I can. So, I ate an apple and sent my blessings off into the universe. And I didn't even reach for the wine.

January 22nd

I am victorious.

If you only focus on where you are today, you can never get to where you want to go. Set a vision for your success and imagine already having it. Claim victory. You are already victorious. Look in the mirror, smile, and say out loud "I am a winner." Try it. You are a winner. You are victorious. Hold your head up and stick your chest out. Stand up and do this now. Raise your hands upward and stretch out your arms.

Claim victory. It's fundamental to your growth to *know* that you can accomplish anything; and then, you accomplish your ultimate goals.

Focus on your winning attitude, your can-do abilities. Leave the doubts behind with practice, the negative gets smaller, the positive becomes all-encompassing, and one day you look up and bam – *victory*.

"Go confidently in the direction of your dreams. Live the life you have imagined." – Henry David Thoreau

January 23rd

I change my body with positive thoughts about eating well.

We want to lose weight, yet when we sit down to eat, we only think about what is delicious or satisfies our craving. The ultimate purpose of food is to nourish our bodies and provide strength and energy. It is completely our own choice on how we think about food. We can choose differently. Turn the channel, close the magazine, and change the conversation.

When we put our attention on thinking more about the vitality of our bodies, rather than our taste buds, we make the choices that create our reality. We are the sum total of our choices. Choices begin with a thought and end with a decision.

Eating well is smart. It is creative. Eating well is world's more satisfying than a fleeting taste on the tongue. It is an enduring energy to carry you throughout the day. Clear eyes, clear head; no pain, no sickness. Think about it... and eat well.

"All that we are is the result of what we have thought."
– Buddha

January 24th

I have peace.

How do you find peace? Is it during a run in a park? Is it when you clean your room? Is it right before you fall asleep?

Find peace within yourself. You have peace, you simply need to lure it out and bring it to life. I find peace within myself when I am still and focused on my presence in the moment. I find peace when my loved ones surround me. I find peace when I'm pursuing my passion for a healthy lifestyle.

Peace is contentment. I know contentment when I choose a spinach salad over the fried chicken sandwich. I'm content when I finish a workout as I feel endorphins rush through my veins. But, I'm content because I know that each decision I make is a positive facet on my wellness journey.

Today, harness that peace. Bring it into each action and each word you speak. Be a beacon of peace today. Bring calm to each person and each situation that greets you.

You have peace. You are peace.

January 25th

Today I see myself the way I want to be.

We each have a vision for ourselves. We creatively borrow the talents or qualities of those we admire, hoping to construct our visions. Whether it's the athleticism, the artistry, or the appearance of our idols, we can occasionally lose sight of the person we want to be.

Today, see yourself the way you want to be. Regard yourself as one of your heroes. Dabble in the hobby of your dreams with courage. Everyone starts out as a beginner, so own your beginner status and participate in each moment with vigor. Instead of lingering on your flaws, direct your attention towards your gifts. Dress today how you'd like to be seen, ranging from sweatpants to a three-piece suit. Vision yourself healthier, livelier, and happier. Inspire yourself. See yourself the way you want to be, and you will become that person. Every action starts with a vision.

January 26th

I practice non-judgment.

Whether you are on a diet or not on a diet, you choose your actions and ultimately choose your future. No one has the authority to judge your diet or lifestyle habits. They do not know what gives you energy or fullness, as you do not know the foods that work best for them. Only you know what's best for your wellness.

Humans are imperfect. It's what separates us from robots, from technology, from boredom. The fun in life comes from adventure, risk-taking, and following your heart (and occasionally, your stomach). It's not always about *what* you eat, but it's about *how* you're eating better.

We each sit in our own cushioned driver seats of life; we are all in charge of our destinies through the decisions we make. You are allowed to eat the candy bar, you're allowed to order a soda, you're allowed to indulge in the bread – but it's the habits of these indulgences that influence your diet odyssey.

Slip up. Make a mistake. You are human. We are not infallible. Don't judge others, don't judge yourself – simply be. Observe. Improve. There will always be potholes, but it's up to you to keep driving.

January 27th

I am happy.

I love moments like these, which turn into days like these, which turn into years like these. These what? Happy moments. What was a good year for you? What made it good and why? You had moments, feelings, emotions, and experiences that created this euphoria we call happiness; you were happy.

Happiness is not elusive. You can capture it at any moment. Like now. Be happy. Think about what you are grateful for. Smile. Recall the last time you laughed until you cried. Put on your favorite fragrance. Take everything people say about you as a compliment today. Find the good in the world. Explore the good in yourself.

My husband regularly reminds me that he spoils me. There was a time I considered spoiled as a negative charactcristic. I worked diligently not to spoil my kids, I wouldn't overspend while shopping and had a thing about being called spoiled. It came from my upbringing. But today, I will give him a big hug and thank him. Yes, I am spoiled. Better yet, I'm blessed… and happy.

January 28th

I am responsible for my life.

Sometimes all we want is a little support from our loved ones, but we must remember to support ourselves. Take time to sit with your decisions & own them. Make sure they are aligned with your life's purpose and don't get easily derailed. Increase your confidence. Encourage yourself.

You can't hold other people accountable for your life because they didn't say what you wanted to hear, in the way you wanted to hear it. Everyone is doing the best they can. Nip the craziness in the bud. You own you. What you wear, your hairstyle, your food choices. Have a party. Or, don't have a party. Don't let people who aren't paying your rent decide your life. Own it, whatever your choice may be. You and you alone are responsible for your life, so find confidence in your decisions, in your actions, in yourself. It's all up to you.

"I am the master of my fate, I am the captain of my soul." -*Invictus,* William Ernest Henley

January 29th

I have mental clarity.

If you could have a superpower, what would you choose? Flight? Invisibility? Reading minds? What if I told you that if you ate a diet of whole foods that you'd gain a superpower? You can, and it's mental clarity. It's not as dazzling as soaring in the night sky or knowing the thoughts of your arch nemesis, but it's astounding what a nutritious diet does to your mind.

You think better, you see better, your attitude improves, you gain the energy to fight crime all night long - that last one might've been a stretch, but nourishing your body with nutrition means cultivating clarity. A clear mind is free from the fog of anxiety, self-hate, or fear. A clear mind initiates each day with a fresh perspective on life. A clear mind is crucial to a positive life.

Eat clean and notice how your memory strengthens, how your mood lightens, and how your wit sharpens.

I have mental clarity.

January 30th

I am focused.

Recall a time in your life where you were focused to achieve a goal and you accomplished it. What did it feel like? Did you think about it all the time? Maybe talk to friends and read about the topic relentlessly?

Retrieve that energy and use it now for your wellness journey. You are focused. You are focused on eating well as a direct route to wellbeing and happiness - and that feels exciting. Focus on this goal. Focus isn't a saying; it's an action.

Select the right groceries. Buy a magazine, subscribe to a daily email, and tune into podcasts that inspire you. Find a support group you can talk to and gain insights & encouragement. This is focus. I like to say maniacal focus, a mad fixation. Concentrate on happy and before you know it, happy will find you. Eat well and be well.

I am healthy.

You have to accept that health is your natural state. Anything unhealthy in your life is the result of an imbalance. It is the result of outside and negative influences that cling to you.

Your mission on your journey to wellbeing is to be aware of those burdens that weigh you down. Peel them back, layer by layer, until your true healthy nature is revealed. Imagine a nut. Pick your favorite. Maybe it's a walnut or a peanut. The healthy you is the nut on the inside of the shell. You want to peel away the hard shell that surrounds the nut. You think it's there to protect you, and while it has served its purpose from time to time, it's your turn to shatter the shell.

Once you crack that outer barrier of unhealthiness, you can grow in your own strength. Your healthy and positive wellbeing makes for a happier life. The shell may protect you, but it's keeping you in darkness. Stuck. Blind. You are healthy. Just break away the shell to experience what fresh air and sunshine truly feel like. It's wellness. It's happy. It's a healthy you.

February 1ˢᵗ

I am persistent.

Persistence is a strong word. To persevere means to continue on even in times of doubt and extreme resistance. It is a pivotal ingredient to success. There is no way around it.

Practice persevering. Don't give up. When decadent food choices present themselves, whether it's the assorted cookies at the gift exchange or the spiked eggnog at the holiday party, repeat this affirmation and move on. Each time you trade that slice of pecan pie for roasted Brussel sprouts, you not only progress towards a healthier diet but also are actively pursuing a healthier life. Take a note from Calvin Coolidge below and press on – to a healthier you.

"Nothing in the world can take the place of persistence. Talent will not; nothing is more common than unsuccessful men with talent. Genius will not; unrewarded genius is almost a proverb. Education will not; the world is full of educated derelicts. Persistence and determination alone are omnipotent. The slogan, 'Press on!' has solved and always will solve the problems of the human race." -Calvin Coolidge

February 2nd

It is my intention to be loving.

Love is a big word. Unfortunately, it's overused and misused to the point where it's lost meaning and ability to stir the most joyous, peaceful, and comforting feeling within us. Today, think about someone you truly love. Reflect on your relationship. Sit with that feeling. Is it your mother, father, or child? A sibling, best friend, mentor, or pet? Whoever it is, close your eyes and think about them.

Turn your attention to this feeling, and its effect on your heart. How does your body feel? Light, strong, or powerful? Do you catch yourself smiling? Is there a pang or flutter of longing encompassing your every move? Feel love. Over time, words failed to convey or describe it really. It's a knowing. A state of being. From there, you show love. You give your best through energy, hugs, and even a reassuring glance. It's not in the gifts or the punctuality or the chores - it's in the heart and body. You don't love fried chicken, cheese crackers, or wine. You love relationships. You love yourself. Elevate love and be intentional.

February 3rd

I eat well so I can be happy.

All anyone really wants is to be happy. For thousands of years, people ask about the formula to joy and success, always looking for a secret weapon or shortcut. Then when you finally reach contentment, you want more – more luxuries, a bigger house, or the next promotion. There is no secret to happiness. The answer isn't hidden; it lives in plain sight, open to all.

Learn to be content with what you have at the present moment. That's it. Simple. Find gratitude in what's right in front of you. You are loved, blessed, and healthy. What you do and appreciate right now will continue to stretch into each moment moving forward. Treat the next moment as you did with this moment. Soon you will find you are content and happy.

Eating well is a crucial building block towards happiness. Eat well this meal, this snack, and this beverage. Each time, the next time, and the times soon to come. You choose to be happy just like how you choose healthy options. You will look up one day after a string of such moments and find happiness. (Hint: happiness is there all along.)

February 4th

I am aware of why I am eating comfort foods.

Why do you eat comfort food? What are your comfort foods? I like peanut butter and jelly sandwiches. They can be gourmet with blackberry preserves or your average store-bought creamy peanut butter and grape jelly (I'm versatile like that). I like peanut butter flavored anything, like Cap'n Crunch® or Reese's Peanut Butter Cups®. Clearly, peanut butter is my comfort go-to.

Why do you eat comfort foods? For comfort, clearly. But if we halt the answer at that point, we'll never get to the real reason. It's always emotionally linked. Dig deep to the root of the issue to know what it is you're comforting, and your comfort food eating will disappear. Why do you eat the specific comfort foods that you choose? I eat what I had as a kid. Growing up, they remind me of my favorite breakfasts, lunches, and after school treats my mom made. It's built off of fond memories and warm feelings. We use food to try and take us to a place. It doesn't work long term.

Why are you eating comfort food?

February 5th

I eat healthy oils.

Not all fats are created equal. The salted, large fry form the drive-thru is not the same as the rich guacamole. Fat doesn't always appear as the bits of your body that you tug from your thighs or belly - fat can be the glow in our skin, the shine in our locks, or the fulfilled feeling after a meal.

Bodies are supposed to have fat because our bodies *need* fat. This type of essential oil aids us in losing weight, maximizes our metabolisms, & coats our hearts with a protective barrier against disease. The good oils and fats to take in on a regular basis are omega-3s from that Alaskan salmon, the monounsaturated fats that give our avocados a smooth texture, and the linoleic acids found in tofu and walnuts.

Embrace the good oils in your life. Don't shun them because they're qualified as fats, but welcome them into your life like the yin to your yang. Create a harmony with these essential fats and open yourself up to the happiness of a well-balanced regimen.

February 6th

I am actively doing the things to create the life I want.

If you want to improve your health or your life, you must actively choose to do so. Manifest the desire for success in each thought and pass on your thoughts to your actions.

Leave your comfort zone to emerge into your dream life and make it a reality through your daily actions. Wake up early, even if you call yourself a night owl. Run a mile, even though you dread cardio. Purchase the package of kale you always avoid and scour magazines for recipes to fit it seamlessly into your diet. Gain an appetite for life. Renew yourself. Urge yourself every day to do something that will catapult you into change. Embody your goals through conscious activity.

Be an active part of your life. Take control of your future by harnessing what you can do in the present. Once you run that first mile, you'll wonder why you haven't started running sooner. Eventually, a healthy lifestyle will become second nature. Reveal your new and improved self, little by little each day.

February 7th

Today I hope to make someone's day better by showing them affection.

I love affection. My kids and I are very affectionate. Apparently too affectionate, according to friends and observers. From their remarks, I learn that everyone wants affection in their own way. The key phrase here is in *their own* way.

There's a growing conversation on love languages. The main concept here is to express love to someone in the way *they* want to be loved, not the way you want to love them. If they are the same, that's great, but most times they are not.

Don't grow angry or upset if your loved one doesn't communicate love the way you do. Maybe they don't like to receive gifts or aren't crazy about physical intimacy like kisses and hugs. It could be based on how they grew up. Maybe they simply want a kind handwritten note or an afternoon of peace & quiet. Maybe a phone call. Make someone's day today. Show them affection how they like it best. Then it's a real gift of love.

February 8th

I make a conscious choice to avoid sugar today.

Sugar is turbo fuel for energy. Like everything, it has a bright side and a shadow. It's sweet and yummy, making your taste buds rejoice with delight. It is also calorie dense, has a quick biochemical reaction in the body, and contributes to weight gain.

Because of the downside, many artificial sweeteners overrule the market. On the bright side, the empty calories are avoided, but a darker shadow of processed by-products are linked to disease.

Work to reduce and eliminate processed sugar from to your diet. Enjoy natural sugar in fruits. Start with one choice at a time. Start today. Choose your wellbeing.

"Great things are done by a series of small things brought together." – Vincent van Gogh

February 9th

I choose love.

It is so much easier to love than to hate. The default setting in this day and age seems to be fear and hate, but that's not true. That's a lie. Choose truth - choose love.

Choosing love is not akin to a one-night stand or a passing affair. You choose love over and over again. I struggle with choosing love when I am confronted with roadblocks or delays from reaching my goals. I find myself wanting to avoid the much needed updates because I fear failure.

But when I am confronted with these roadblocks, I choose love. I choose to expect the best, not prepare for the worst. I realize I attract the delays by believing there will be delays. I create problems where there aren't any.

If you meet a delay in your journey or a prolonged red light, look at it from a positive point of view and choose love. Expect success today, regardless. It's for your own good. Love is always for your own good. Choose love.

February 10th

I am worthy.

The universe and your higher power joined forces to craft you – isn't that absolutely magical? Together, they divvied up duties delicately picking out your features, choosing your talents, and designing you to reflect the great wonders beyond this world.

You are worthy. You are worthy of the spirit, the mentality, and the body you want. You are worthy of life fully lived because you *have* a life. Take pride in the fact that you are alive and breathing. You are a walking miracle.

Know your value. Value is not based on the opinions of others but curated from your uniqueness. No one on this entire planet is like you. They might resemble you, talk like you, or dress like you, but none possess your rare talents.

To find your own worth, you must embrace your uniqueness, quirks and all. Your individuality leads to the grand discovery of self-worth.

February 11th

I choose to eat whole foods today.

The more you eat food that is closer to its natural state, the healthier you will be. Today, make conscious choices to eat fruits, vegetables, rice, and beans. Avoid processed foods like artificially flavored energy bars or sugary breakfast cereals. The additives weaken your immune system, keeping your weight clocked in on overtime.

Imagine yourself as a cavewoman or caveman; your only goal is to stay alive. The ancient man ate from the earth and those who follow the Paleo diet attempt to reach back to the origins of man. Whole, fresh foods are the foundation to build upon your healthy lifestyle. You will find the more you eat from the Earth, like the first of mankind to walk the Earth, the stronger you become. And you can't dispute that, these people ran alongside wild animals, hunting for food.

Choose whole foods, not processed, and cork the bottle of wine. When you wake up tomorrow, take note of how you feel. When you practice this day on more and more days, you'll see your energy and willpower grow to new heights.

February 12th

Today I will examine my relationships for healing.

Do a scan of all of your relationships. Do it quickly because typically, your first thought or feeling is your most honest. Start with each member in your household. Expand to your family living outside your home, your best friends, your work relationships, your community, neighbors and so on. At least scan the top 10 people you associate with regularly.

Do you gain a warm, fuzzy, loving feeling? Supportive? Or is there fear and anxiety? Do you feel like an outsider or judge, or like a friend and companion? Create a conscious note of who is supporting you to become the best you can be. Sometimes when you start to glow and exude confidence, those people who you thought were on your team start to turn their back on you. Recognize if you are doing this to someone in your life and make a better change.

Start today by spending more time with the positive people. Those are the healing relationships. The others? Well, you know.

February 13th

My true self is valuable beyond measure.

It would be impossible to calculate how many lives you've touched. Your mere existence has meaning far beyond yourself. We often think about those special people who touched our lives, but rarely think about the lives we have touched.

The nurses and doctors at the hospital you were born in, your parents, siblings, cousins, neighbors, friends, and teachers are just the initial list of people you have impacted. In the grocery store, movies, airplanes or the bus, even the post office – people everywhere are impacted by your energy, smile, and grace.

You bring your full self to every experience and encounter. You are monumental. Powerful. Outstandingly valuable.

"Wherever you go, there you are." – Ram Dass

February 14th

I am loved.

You are not alone. You are loved. God loves you, I love you, and people that don't even know you love you. Love isn't only reserved for your significant other or your family. Love is in everything. Love is in the smiles from strangers, the tears at a wedding or a funeral. Love is in the birds singing and the droplets of rain. Love is compassion and caring - the sincerest expressions.

You are loved. Not only are you loved simply because you're you, but you are an expression of love. You *are* love. It's time you know your worth. Understand that there are so few words to describe or define love. It's too grand; it's all-encompassing. Words barely scratch the surface of the concept. Because to truly know love, you have to feel it. Feel it with your soul. Not just the 5 senses you're used to.

When you see love in everything, you recognize its home in yourself. You cherish yourself and you share it freely with others. You are loved. You are love.

February 15th

I take three deep breaths when I am stressed and want to turn to food.

We eat to nourish our bodies and gain energy to make it through the day. We also eat as a filler - to fill an emptiness within us, emotionally, spiritually, mentally, or physically. You control your next moment and decide how you will handle your stress. Some turn to cigarettes or alcohol. The most commonly accepted form, and most overlooked, is food. Only you control what you eat. No one can monitor your limit but yourself. You have the power. It is difficult to control habits that have been built up over a lifetime. Years ago, I picked up the habit of smoking. And I won't lie; I enjoyed it immensely in the moment. But when I realized the toll on my health and the resulting long-term issues, I quit one cigarette at a time. With a dedication to change and a yearning for a healthier life, I found my breath again.

Breathe into your stress. Run your stress away. Talk your stresses out with a trusted ear. Don't eat your stress. Respect the beautiful growth of a healthy routine replacing a lazy habit.

February 16th

Today I bless my knees.

Thank you, knees, for being and keeping a steady rhythm with my thoughts and actions. I think of ropes and pulleys, slides, hinges, swing sets, seesaws and a world of physics when I think of how you function. Simple, yet mysterious.

I smile to myself when I imagine legs without knees. Everything would be straight. I know you are left sick sometimes from the wear and tear of standing, walking, and sports. I put a lot of weight on you and don't give you credit for all you do. With a balanced diet, I hope to decrease some of that weight and allow you to regain your energy.

Thank you, knees. I will be kinder to you today.

February 17th

I have integrity.

Integrity is the quality of being honest and having strong moral principles - a gut feeling of moral uprightness. Integrity is what you have to do even when no one is looking and there is no reward. Too often in this world, people compromise their integrity for a short-term benefit. You'll reap out of this world what you put into it. If you abide by the laws of karma, you recognize what goes around comes back around.

Make your choices openly and in your best and highest values. Solidify your actions based on that karmic evolution. Usually the hardest decisions have the highest integrity, but you reap the biggest rewards.

Even if it's as simple as forgiving a friend or apologizing for a fault, once you act with integrity, positivity will cascade into your life with the power of a surging river. The other day my taxes haunted me in my sleep. But I would not be moving down the righteous path of integrity to close my eyes and flee, so I paid what was owed. Instantly, happiness flooded me as I slipped the check in the mailbox. Burden gone. Amazing.

Time is a great healer.

Time heals all wounds both big and small. While may leave scars, the wound heals. Whatever the tragedy, the healing becomes a part of you. A scar, which changes color and shape over time, heals to become thicker than the original skin. Time changes you through an evolving perspective. You mature while growing stronger and wiser.

In the moment, circumstances can appear more complicated than they truly are. We as humans jump to conclusions and search for problems. We think up all the different ways something can go wrong, without seeing the ways it can go right.

Today, appreciate the time. Through the passing of time, you grow. You struggle because growth is uncomfortable (they don't call them "growing pains" for nothing). To be comfortable means you choose not to challenge yourself.

Know that achieving wellness and health isn't an overnight process. You won't see results tomorrow morning. But, if you work every day, you will find wellbeing. Time will tell. It always does.

I order appetizers for my meal and share entrees.

Portion sizes at restaurants in the Americanized culture are grandiose. If there's an option to super-size your meal, resist the urge. These mega-sized portions are often doubled what is considered normal. It takes you back to the times when you thought you had a balanced or healthy meal, when in reality, you may have consumed a significant amount of calories, overdoing what your body needed.

When you venture to a hip new restaurant or stop for a bite along a road trip, be portion prepared. Ask about portion sizes. Rarely ever do you need an appetizer *and* a meal. In European countries, appetizers are petite and made for sharing amongst large groups. In the United States, ordering an appetizer likens to another entrée. Are you questioning a fried appetizer, say calamari or mozzarella sticks? That's calorie and fat dense. Getting a 16 oz. steak? The average portion is four ounces per serving. Surprised at how much you're eating? Now you know.

Share an entrée or stop after the appetizer. It's all you really need.

February 20th

I eat bread sparingly.

Bread is magnificent. But not just any loaf wrapped in cellophane, the type of bread that cracks when you push the crust with intricate holes of chewy dough. Like anything in this world, bread is only good in moderation. It's not very realistic to purchase the fresh French loaf daily. But on those special occasions, with an appetizer board of delicacies, then good bread becomes great.

Today, eat bread sparingly. If your body or metabolism needs carbs, slip in a slice of bread during your morning breakfast or afternoon lunch to utilize those carbs as energy. Capitalize on the carbs for your workday; work them off throughout the evening.

Make bread something you can look forward to, not something you have with each meal. Eat your toast with heart-healthy avocado or fresh fruit to prolong your morning activity. Bite into the roll with your salad if need be. Don't over-exercise the role of bread in your diet. Only bring out the big guns when necessary.

February 21ˢᵗ

I practice selflessness.

I never understood the phrase, "the reason you don't get along with so-and-so is because you are so much alike." I love myself — if we adhere to that logic, we should have great chemistry together like a couple of snow peas in a pod.

Take a minute to think about someone who annoys you and examine why. When you become aware of what you are judging, and why you are judging, you can release that negative energy. Self-discovery is like a yogurt parfait. The more you dig in, the more you're greeted with new flavors, both soft and strong, about yourself. Sometimes you're even delightfully surprised.

Be selfless by not allowing what others do to interfere with your harmony. That is not selfish, but *selfless*. It means you don't put your values on someone else. Every story has two narrators. Even when it's cloudy outside, the sun still shines behind the clouds. When you decide to break the heavy chains of judgment that causes fear, you free yourself to achieve anything. You have the key. Unlock the shackles. Be selfless to others and you will ultimately soar.

February 22nd

I am positive and that positive energy is received and comes back to me effortlessly.

Positive thinking is a magnet for positive results. The energy around you reacts to your thinking. Everything begins with a thought. If you think something enough, you start to believe it. And when you think positive, happy, excited thoughts, then that energy will become positive.

Your aura adapts to what you release into the world. It flows around you constantly and reflects your attitude. I'm sure you could name one person you know who is notably joyous. They take on each day of life and search for the cheerful moments. And, like a magnet, they attract those moments back into their lives. They're encircled by positivity.

You get what you give. What you put out into the world, even with one passing thought, will come back into your life. Release positivity and positivity will return in the most unexpected and enchanting way.

February 23rd

Gratitude allows me to harness the positive energy to eat well.

Often we eat as a filler for some emptiness or disappointment. We have our go-to comfort foods or our favorite bottle of wine. It slows us down, mellows us out, and we sip our glasses of Cabernet believing it's a good thing. And it can be if it is celebratory or for a much-needed vacation, but it shouldn't evolve into your nightly rituals. Everything that glitters isn't gold; if every night you eat your family size bag of cheese puffs or down the three glasses of wine, your wellness journey becomes clouded with fog and thunderstorms.

A much greater way to fill the emptiness is with a practice of gratitude. Comfort is the feeling you are going for when you over-eat. Next time when you are looking for comfort or respite from stress or loneliness, take time to bask in your blessings and ponder what you are grateful for. Marvel in how you are grateful for your health and your journey to improved wellbeing.

Today you can harness comfort gratitude, instead of comfort food, to eat well and design a better path to overall happiness.

February 24th

I will stretch my legs once an hour.

Stretching is underrated. Have you ever stood up from your desk or couch, reached your hands over your head, and exhaled out stress as you dove towards your toes? It's a feeling of calm that rushes over your skin like a wave as you feel the blood traveling through your veins. Flickers of light pop up in your eyesight to remind you you're alive.

When you stretch, you energize your body. Substitute the mid-day coffee break for a revitalizing stretch session. Increase the blood flow to your body without the caffeine crash. The more you stretch, the more in-tune you are with your body. Your loose limbs will mean less pain and you'll adapt the proper form needed for exercising, finally achieving that perfect form needed to maximize the results of your workout.

Stretching is stress relief. Relieve your muscles while mentally stretching your mind. Relax into the stretch without straining yourself. Take a few minutes throughout the day today to find those peaceful moments.

February 25th

I realize that sauces, dressing, and oils have hidden calories.

The thick, white texture of ranch dressing doesn't exactly come off as low-carb. With a base of buttermilk and high sodium, the fatty ranch dressing does not add any nutritional value to your veggies. When people transition into salads, they sometimes reach towards unhealthier dressing options to make the bowl of greens as appetizing as a deluxe pizza. But the more we add thick dressings or oils high in trans fats, we take away the nutritional benefit from the salad itself. Creamy Alfredo sauce and Thousand Island dressing are high in fats. Caesar dressing isn't too far off either, with the amount of cheese and oil that make up its savory taste.

We all need to dress up our plates sometimes, and that's where dressings come into play. If you need to top off your plate with a little something extra, opt for oil and vinegar over the pre-portioned Italian dressing. You can control your oil intake, which helps you save calories, and vinegar, whether it's balsamic or apple cider, gives it that tanginess you desire.

You can avoid fatty dressings today – awaken your creativity for healthier options.

February 26th

I focus on eliminating the cause of my disease.

Society portrays quick cures for everything; too many people search for hasty remedies in pills or surgery. Eat too much? Swoop up the pack of diet pills or a belly wrap. Maybe consult for a surgery to staple your stomach. Have a chronic condition caused by too much sodium? Take a blood pressure pill. Diabetes? We now have hospital wings dedicated to this prolific condition.

Start looking towards the causes of these conditions. Work to change these and see amazing results. Diet and exercise. Read it aloud: *diet and exercise.* As surely as these solutions cure the adversaries that promote our sicknesses, the lack of proper diet and exercise is often the culprit for the condition.

Incorporate a low glycemic diet. Eat whole foods. Eliminate pesticides, bad bacteria, and inflammatory foods. Delve to ground zero and eliminate the problem at the source. Don't wait on a pill.

February 27th

My priorities are aligned with my actions.

What are your priorities? List your top three. Here are some common ones: 1. God, country, family. 2. God, family, career. 3. Family, friends, career. 4. Health, career, family.

This list can endlessly trail on and on with possibilities. The point is, you live a happier life when the places you spend your time and your actions align with your priorities. Do you put God first, yet spend little or no time in prayer, praise, or gratitude? Is family first, but the last time you attended a family dinner was too distant to remember?

Decide the priorities you want to have in your life. Not what society says, but what's in your heart. Is it service to others? Is it finding shelter for the homeless? Being a CEO? Raising a happy family? Make a list. Then make a list next to it in the order of where you spend your time.

Alter your life to add and deduct time, bringing these lists in alignment. Stress is misalignment. Happiness, however, is a perfect fit.

February 28th

Today I focus on eating nutritious foods.

It's challenging to focus on some type of restriction when trying to eat well or lose weight. Low calorie, low carb, low whatever. When you focus on the lack, what you receive is restrictions. It is difficult to achieve wellness when you focus on what you cannot have.

Today, concentrate on what you can have. Spin it positively. Put your mind on what vegetables and fruits are in season and find a tasty way to have them in a meal. Fixate on nutritious foods, not only the foods that fit into a calorie count. It's far too easy to like unhealthy, processed foods, compensating for a calorie count.

Focus on the spirit of eating well. Eat nutritiously.

February 29th

Your full potential rests in your hands.

Just like my choices have infinite possibilities, so do the outcomes. Listen to the stories of successful leaders, entrepreneurs, or visionaries. Some come from slums, others come from trust funds; some accredit God to their success, while others simply went to work every day.

You have infinite possibilities in your life to create health, happiness, and wealth, no matter your circumstances. Initially, you must recognize and believe this is true. Then you make the choices. Just one at a time will do, however small. Most people hand over the power to fear, afraid that they are not good enough, or unprepared, or unworthy. You are worthy. And you can only be prepared by taking each step and challenge that comes before you. Infinity, eternity, immortality, enlightenment - you got this.

Create the life you want. Be healthy, happy, and wise.

"The only person you are destined to become is the person you decide to be." -Ralph Waldo Emerson

Epilogue

I hope these affirmations have filled you with inspiration and touched your life, just as they've influenced mines. With these goals, I could set an intention for how to positively think, act, and live throughout my day. These hopeful reminders were designed to help me stay on track and focus on my health and wellbeing while integrating all areas of my life into my wellness journey- family, career, and everything in between.

These daily affirmations inspired me in ways beyond what I fed myself each day. It started with adding more vegetables to my diet, to sharing my leftovers with others, and soon to cultivating a life of pride and self-love. As I practiced mindfulness and internalized these affirmations, before I knew it I was following my true purpose…practicing and sharing mindfulness as a path to wellbeing. I embraced my hidden entrepreneurial energy and created UGottaEat, a smartphone app to connect people and their communities through food. I never expected that with each simple objective for the day, my life would be impacted so greatly.

I share my personal pilgrimage with you because my results have been so profound. Every day begins with a thought that transfers to an emotion. This emotion will dictate your day, your month, and your life.

Calming inspiration is empowering. I found through these declarations a discovery of self. I started to sleep better, stress less, walk more, be present, and of course, eat mindfully. With each passing day and each written affirmation, I actively created a healthier, happier me. I find balance.

Allow the affirmations that make up this book to act as a guiding force to help you better define what health means to you. Discover your version of wellbeing. Take liberty with these affirmations. They are not rules carved into stone, but ideas that flow through the air like leaves in the wind. Allow them to touch your soul and internalize them. Find the methods that work for your personal wellbeing.

I hope you continue to find a healthier, happier you through each statement, question, and affirmation. I send my love, light, and blessings to you. Eat well. Live well. Be well.

UGottaEat...So Eat Mindfully.

Index

every day; **Page 308** I believe and declare I am everything God created me to be; **Page 310** The scale only has the power that I give it to change my mood; **Page 324** I am eating for my wellbeing more and eating out of habit less; **Page 335** I am prepared; **Page 351** I am victorious; **Page 353** I have peace; **Page 354** Today I see myself the way I want to be; **Page 360** I am healthy; **Page 370** I am worthy; **Page 371** I choose to eat whole foods today; **Page 377** I have integrity; **Page 382** I am positive and that positive energy is received and comes back to me effortlessly

If you need motivation or a sense of direction, turn to: Page 19 Today I expand my awareness; **Page 36** I make decisions from positive emotions; **Page 49** I choose abundance; **Page 52** I am visualizing my success; **Page 60** When I let go, I gain everything; **Page 74** I am visioning my life as I want it to be; **Page 82** I am consistent; **Page 104** My beliefs filter my experiences; **Page 116** In every moment, I can choose from infinite possibilities; **Page 129** I ask my higher power to order my steps; **Page 134** I am living in the present moment; **Page 141** My positive choices create a chain reaction toward my goals; **Page 145** I connect with people who improve and motivate me; **Page 153** I am able to break old habits and create new ones; **Page 161** I am worth the effort; **Page 164** I am in charge of my beliefs and choices; **Page 176** I am transforming my life; **Page 207** I am right where I am supposed to be;

Page 213 I create my own success every day; **Page 221** I acknowledge there is a higher power offering me guidance; **Page 225** I trust my intuition; **Page 237** I activate the possible; **Page 255** I connect with my true self; **Page 282** When challenges arise, I ask myself, "What can I learn from this?"; **Page 292** My outlook filters what I see; **Page 329** My goals align with my spirit; **Page 330** I am motivated; **Page 334** I can only change what I am aware of; **Page 339** I am disciplined; **Page 342** Success is not determined by the brilliance of my plan, but by the consistency of my actions; **Page 343** I am the master of my fate; **Page 350** I get things done when I fixate my full attention on my goal; **Page 358** I have mental clarity; **Page 359** I am focused; **Page 361** I am persistent; **Page 366** I am actively doing the things to create the life I want; **Page 378** Time is a great healer; **Page 387** My priorities are aligned with my actions

If you could use a little inspiration, turn to: Page 38 I humble myself; **Page 42** I love life; **Page 99** I am powerful; **Page 101** I believe that God and those who love me accept me for who I am; **Page 103** I am important; **Page 110** I am in harmony; **Page 115** I am blessed with a new vision for my life; **Page 121** I am excited; **Page 128** I am empowered; **Page 132** I am unapologetically me; **Page 143** I have courage; **Page 170** I am supported by my friends and neighbors; Page 174** I am powerful. I matter. I make a difference. ; **Page**

179 I am strong; **Page 197** Today I give myself permission to be free; **Page 202** I am an influencer; **Page 204** I recognize my potential is unlimited; & so it is; **Page 229** I am free to express my authentic true self; **Page 244** I am resilient; **Page 259** I am my biggest supporter; **Page 269** My quality of life improves every day; **Page 274** I am accepting; **Page 299** I am blessed; **Page 312** I am generous; **Page 314** I understand that only light can dissolve darkness; **Page 325** I have joy; **Page 336** My spiritual true self and my worldly self are congruent; **Page 347** I am courageous; **Page 348** I am complete; **Page 356** I am happy; **Page 373** My true self is valuable beyond measure; **Page 374** I am loved; **Page 389** Your full potential rests in your hands

If you want to focus more on your food, turn to:
Page 20 I am eating purposefully; **Page 32** I plan what I will eat for the week; **Page 37** I take three deep breaths when I feel upset and want a drink; **Page 47** I wait 5 minutes and examine why I am having a craving and make a conscious decision; **Page 51** I make the conscious choice to drink alcohol only when I have pre-planned my eating choices; **Page 54** I focus on my food while I am eating; **Page 63** I choose portion sizes that align with the level of health and wellness I desire; **Page 84** I acknowledge that moderation is the key to eating and drinking well; **Page 100** I recognize the emotional triggers that make me want to eat more; **Page 120** I read books and magazines that promote health; **Page**

caffeine today; **Page 344** I pack my lunch the day before; **Page 375** I take three deep breaths when I am stressed and want to turn to food; **Page 379** I order appetizers for my meal and share entrees.

If you want a beautiful relationship with food, turn to: **Page 40** I will do something different today to shake things up and break my "habit" neuron pathways; **Page 41** I take time to enjoy the color of the foods on my plate; **Page 46** Eating Well + Awareness = Happiness; **Page 62** I have a positive relationship with food; **Page 107** I eat well because it gives me confidence; **Page 154** I perform at peak condition; **Page 175** I am aware that healthful eating leads to a healthy life and vitality; **Page 178** I improve my life by making conscious choices to eat well; **Page 239** I eat healthfully for peak performance; **Page 248** I am aware that a whole foods diet improves my wellbeing; **Page 281** I utilize healthy dinner sharing and sharing with my friends and neighbors for convenience and wellness; **Page 287** I am eating slowly today to enjoy my food more; **Page 291** I eat well because it nourishes me; **Page 315** I have constant access to healthy foods to increase my wellness; **Page 332** Eating well makes me feel good about my choices; **Page 363** I eat well so I can be happy; **Page 388** Today I focus on eating nutritious foods

If you want motivation to eat well, turn to: **Page 23** I make choices that improve my life one meal at a time; **Page 44** I will go to a fresh new market; **Page 57** I wait 5 minutes before I satisfy a sweet and salty craving; **Page 68** I am making at least one conscious choice to avoid processed food today; **Page 75** Today I focus on fiber; **Page 78** I eat well to have energy for my friends; **Page 81** I keep healthy food choices handy; **Page 97** I make a conscious choice to avoid fatty foods; Page **109** I eat food made from scratch; **Page 114** I am reinventing myself into the person I always wanted to be; **Page 133** I eat fruit as a snack today; **Page 144** I eat only one dessert this week; **Page 149** I drink non-alcoholic beverages today; Page **158** I eat fresh made food; **Page 169** I eat my last meal at least two hours before I sleep; **Page 193** I will monitor my salt intake today; **Page 199** I eat homemade food; **Page 210** I am prepared for tomorrow; **Page 215** I eat well to give thanks to the universe; **Page 230** I spend more time on the outside grocery store aisles; **Page 233** My food is medicine to my body; **Page 245** I acknowledge that unhealthy eating leads to low energy and chronic diseases; **Page 249** I fill nighttime snacking with fresh vegetables and fruits; **Page 252** I will replace ordering dessert with a nice warm cup of coffee or tea; **Page 262** Today I focus on healthy fats; **Page 276** I eat healthful carbs today; **Page 283** I eat well to have energy for my family; **Page 294** I use sauces and dressings sparingly; **Page 301** I eat homemade food more than I eat out; **Page 304** I wait 5 minutes before I satisfy a craving for fast food to give myself time to make the best choice for me; **Page 309** Today I focus on protein; **Page 313** This week I will have salad at least one meal per day; **Page 327** I am eating only fruits and vegetables today; **Page 337** I will subscribe to a wellness blog; **Page 340** I eat only 1 serving which is enough to nourish me; **Page 346** I am buying healthful foods today in preparation for eating healthy later this week; **Page 349** I maximize my metabolism by eating well; **Page 365** I eat healthy oils; **Page 368** I make a conscious choice to avoid sugar today; **Page 380** I eat bread sparingly; **Page 385** I realize that sauces, dressing, and oils have hidden calories

If you want to focus on your body, turn to: Page 26 I recognize that rest is an important part of vitality; **Page 85** I have more energy and vitality when I eat well; **Page 87** I bring loving attention to my kidneys today; **Page 90** I will chew each bite of food 15-20 times; **Page 93** I spend more time outside with nature which calms my mood and keeps my appetite satisfied; **Page 105** I will walk today; **Page 117** I bring loving attention to my liver today; **Page 124** I walk 30 minutes daily; **Page 125** Today I bless my arms; **Page 130** I stay hydrated; **Page 136** I park a conscious distance away so I can walk more; **Page 155** Today I bless my butt; **Page 162** I bring loving attention to my arteries today; **Page 163** I am healing my body by eating well; **Page 180** Today I bless my thighs and quadriceps, which power my stability; **Page 196** I sleep well because I wind down for bedtime; **Page 211** I bring loving attention to my lungs today; **Page 218** Today I bless my chest; **Page 219** I organize my daily activity to ensure I have enough sleep; **Page 226** I walk to destinations less than one mile away; **Page 279** Today I bless my back; **Page 305** Today I bless and appreciate my stomach that does a wonderful job digesting the food I put in it; **Page 311** I substitute positive activities for my nighttime habit of snacking; **Page 326** I walk up stairs more every day; **Page 376** Today I bless my knees; **Page 384** I will stretch my legs once an hour

If it's intention you're after, turn to: Page 55 It is my intention to be healthy; **Page 126** It is my intention to have an alert mind; **Page 189** I am intentional about what I want; **Page 234** It is my intention to eat well; **Page 238** It is my intention to be a positive role model for others; It is my intention to let my inner strength be a beacon for others; **Page 258** It is my intention to live fully; **Page 362** It is my intention to be loving.

If you hope to exude compassion, turn to: Page 71 I feel good that eating well enlivens me and helps the environment; **Page 77** Gratitude allows me to have compassion for others; **Page 89** I am compassionate; **Page 157** Today I send silent blessings to those who struggle with their body image, for they are me; **Page 212** I am giving focus and attention today to my positive features and being thankful; **Page 228** Today I celebrate my friend's victories with them; **Page 242** My spirit is contagious; **Page 254** Relationships are important to eat healthy; **Page 261** I make thoughtful decisions; **Page 268** I am beneath no one and superior to no one; **Page 273** I practice humility; **Page 275** I am a positive influence on my community; **Page 293** Today I make someone else's day better by acknowledging them; **Page 307** I practice compassion; **Page 341** I remind myself that others have the same issues that I do; **Page 355** I practice non-judgment; **Page 367** Today I hope to make someone's day better by showing them affection.

If you desire to serve yourself and others, turn to: **Page 24** I take responsibility for my life; **Page 48** I support local cooks and chefs who support my goal to eat well; **Page 66** I adopt the habits of people that surround me; **Page 79** I practice non-resistance; **Page 118** I overcome the struggles of my health journey by helping others; **Page 148** It is my intention to serve; **Page 200** I understand that fear is false evidence appearing real; **Page 208** I am constantly learning and evolving; **Page 215** Today I celebrate my victories big and small; **Page 220** I take time to be still and feel the divine energy that is within me; **Page 224** I am building relationships with others who also want to eat healthy and to be happy; **Page 236** I practice non-attachment; **Page 246** I believe everyone should have access to fresh and homemade food; **Page 266** I recognize that I create my self-image and it is positive; **Page 277** I eat only what I need and share what I cannot consume; **Page 285** I am influencing healthier eating habits for my friends and family; **Page 290** I am happy to share my meals with other families; **Page 295** Today I will slow down enough to let peace catch up with me and protect me from choices made under stress; **Page 300** I have positive relationships that support my wellbeing; **Page 317** I am happy to benefit from foods my friends share with me; **Page 331** I find my true self in stillness; **Page 372** Today I will examine my relationships for healing.

If you seek gratitude, turn to: **Page 27** I am grateful; **Page 65** Homemade = Happiness; **Page 88** I take time to enjoy the smell of food; **Page 113** Gratitude + Forgiveness = Love; **Page 119** I am thankful for the weather today; **Page 122** I am thankful for my local grocer; **Page 146** I acknowledge we are all connected; **Page 172** I am kind to the earth for providing sustenance; **Page 183** I am thankful for my safety; **Page 194** I take time to enjoy the taste of each bite; **Page 203** I recognize the magnitude of conditions that must work in harmony to make each meal possible; **Page 227** I take time to enjoy the texture of each bite; **Page 231** I recognize the role that the earth plays in providing the food on my plate; **Page 251** I give thanks for the farmers who harvest the food; **Page 271** Gratitude is the magical key to happiness; **Page 288** I am inspired by my positive relationships; **Page 289** I am thankful;

Page 303 I give thanks for each meal before I eat it; **Page 321** Gratitude allows me to accentuate my positivity; **Page 328** I express gratitude every day; **Page 323** Gratitude allows me to harness the positive energy I need to receive grace; **Page 383** Gratitude allows me to harness the positive energy to eat well.

If you're looking a real eye-opener, for mind, body, and spirit, turn to: **Page 28** I am making a major change today to reflect my enthusiasm for higher wellbeing; **Page 30** I am what I eat; **Page 33** I bring loving attention to my heart today; **Page 43** My thoughts have the power to change lives; **Page 45** I recognize that the pain in my body is a call to action; **Page 50** I choose joy; **Page 59** I understand that others' opinions are a reflection of them and not me; **Page 61** Today I bless my waistline and give thanks for the early warning signs it provides me; **Page 67** I am aware that my thoughts control my emotions; **Page 70** I am aware that sugar is addictive; **Page 73** I am aware that excessive body weight can lead to chronic diseases; **Page 94** I am aware that restaurants use techniques that cause weight gain; **Page 123** I eat fast food strategically; **Page 131** I am imagining my healthier body in the future; **Page 142** Today I honor my body as a temple; **Page 147** I change my body, by changing how I think about my body; **Page 187** I choose harmony; **Page 192** I recognize that my body is my container; **Page 241** I recognize society focuses on quick fixes; **Page 265** I am aware of the importance of rest; **Page 272** I recognize that eating well is the best medicine for the body; **Page 296** I choose mental satisfaction over physical satisfaction; **Page 319** I am aware that sugar contributes to inflammation in my body; **Page 322** I choose peace; **Page 345** I bring loving attention to my skin today; **Page 352** I change my body with positive thoughts about eating well; **Page 369** I choose love; **Page 386** I focus on eliminating the cause of my disease.

If you desire to find a sense of purpose through positive opportunities, turn to: **Page 31** I will satisfy my cravings with healthy choices; **Page 34,** I practice mindful eating; **Page 38** I am supported by others who enjoy a lifestyle of wellness; **Page 64** I recognize that anything worth having is worth waiting for; **Page 76** My motives for eating well align with my highest and best values; **Page 86** I burst the myth that eating healthy is more expensive; **Page 92** I practice forgiveness; **Page 98** I share my wellness affirmations with others who want encouragement; **Page 151** My thoughts choose what I will eat today; **Page 165** I eat foods from local cooks and chefs; **Page 198** My positive thoughts will create positive outcomes; **Page 209** I am aware that mimosas and Bloody Mary's are not actually breakfast foods; **Page 253** I practice patience; **Page 284** I practice kindness; **Page 338** When I am bored, I find productive ways to fill that void and maintain healthful eating habits; **Page 357** I am responsible for my life;

Acknowledgement of Quotes

Throughout this book of daily affirmations, I have placed quotes and mentions of intelligent women and men, as well as notable scripture. These influential people throughout history have acted as a source of my inspiration. Hopefully, they can help you with their words of wisdom, too. I would like to thank these notable icons for motivating fresh thought and captivating ideas in my own wellness journey.

A Year of ME

Albert Einstein

Alice Walker

Aristotle

Bill Gates

Bob Marley

Buddha

Calvin Coolidge

C.S. Lewis

Dalai Lama

Dante Alighieri

Eckhart Tolle

Edward Smith-Stanley

Eleanor Roosevelt

Gandhi

Gary Zukov

Henry David Thoreau

Heraclitus

The Holy Bible

James Allen

Lao Tzu

Lewis Grizzard

Lewis Smedes

Lucille Ball

Martin Luther King Jr.

Maya Angelou

Michael Jackson

Mother Theresa

Napoleon Hill

Oprah Winfrey

Plutarch

Ralph Ellison

Ralph Waldo Emerson

Ram Dass

Robert Urich

Rumi

Seneca the Younger

Socrates

Steve Jobs

Susan Elizabeth Phillips

Thomas Edison

Thomas Jefferson

Vincent van Gogh

Virginia Woolf

William Ernest Henley

Winston Churchill

CPSIA information can be obtained
at www.ICGtesting.com
Printed in the USA
FFOW03n0220071217
43931442-43006FF